Attitudes Toward Post-Menopausal Women In The High And Late Middle Ages, 1100-1400

Attitudes Toward Post-Menopausal Women In The High And Late Middle Ages, 1100-1400

Jessica E. Godfrey

To order additional copies of this book, contact:
Xlibris Corporation
1-888-795-4274
www.Xlibris.com
Orders@Xlibris.com
97142

For the history professors at SUNY Oswego, thank you.

Cover Image: "The Old Woman" by Hans Holbein from *The Dance of Death* (1538).

CONTENTS

INTRODUCTION

Very little has been written about the aged in the Middle Ages and even less on old women. The study of life stages in history is a relatively new topic in the field of history. Historians have only recently (about thirty years ago) begun writing in detail about this subject. Their investigation of life stages in history have been influenced by fields such as biology, psychology, anthropology, and sociology. However, the topic of post-menopausal women has not received much attention in historical scholarship. This may be due to a lack of interest and/or primary sources on the topic.

Sources concerning the elderly in pre-industrial Europe have primarily concentrated on men. The few exceptions are Michael Sheehan's *Aging and the Aged in Medieval Europe* (1983), Georges Minois' *History of Old Age* (1987), Shulamith Shahar's *Growing Old in the Middle Ages* (1995), and Albrecht Classen's *Old Age in the Middle Ages and the Renaissance: Interdisciplinary Approaches to a Neglected Topic* (2007).

Attitudes Toward Post-Menopausal Women in the High and Late Middle Ages, 1100-1400, examines and evaluates didactic and prescriptive sources (religious, philosophical, and medical), literary sources (poems, plays, and literature), and evidence of lived lives (court records, wills, tax and coroners' rolls, and chronicles) in regard to post-menopausal women during the High and Late Middle Ages in England, France, Germany, the Low Countries, and Italy. It analyzes some of the attitudes and perceptions held by medieval writers concerning post-menopausal women. Moreover, it looks at whether discourses on post-menopausal women reflected or diverged from how they actually lived their lives.

The book begins in 1100 with the Crusades, the growth of cities, the appearance of universities, the re-emergence of Greek works in Western Europe from Arabic translations, the increase of heretical sects, and the rise of Church power. It concludes in 1400, before the surge of witchcraft accusations and trials in Europe. A combination of economic and environmental problems, along with misogyny, may have led to women serving as scapegoats during the Witchcraze.[1]

It is difficult, if not impossible, to come up with an exact age at which a woman was considered old in the Middle Ages. Sources either had diverse views on the subject or excluded women altogether. Following Greek, Roman, and Muslim tradition, medieval authors categorized people into age groups. Dividing life into stages was common in a variety of medieval texts: medical, didactic, and literary. During the thirteenth century, writings on the stages of life reached a broader audience as more works appeared in the vernacular. In these texts, life was typically divided into three, four, six, or seven stages. The division of life into three stages was based on Aristotelian biology, the division into four stages on physiology and nature (i.e. the four seasons, four elements, four humors), the division into six stages on the biblical scheme of St. Augustine of Hippo, and the division into seven stages on astrology following Ptolemy.[2]

Medieval writers held similar and distinct views on when old age began. The scientific encyclopedias, *De Natura Rerum* (*On the Nature of Things*, c.1228-40) by Thomas de Cantimpré, *De Rerum Proprietatibus* (*On the Properties of Things*, c.1230-40) by Bartholomaeus Anglicus, and *Speculum Naturale* (*Mirror of Nature*, 1244-54) by Vincent de Beauvais, stated that old age began at fifty. In Aldebrandin of Siena's medical treatise, *Le Régime du Corps* (*The Regimen of the Body*, c.1256-57), he wrote that old age commenced at forty, while Philip de Novare's didactic treatise, *Les Quatre Ages de l'Homme* (*The Four Ages of Man*, c.1260), asserted that it started at sixty. In Dante Alighieri's book of verse, *Il Convivio* (*The Banquet*, c.1304-07), he believed that old age began at forty-five, while Bernard de Gordon's medical work, *De Conservatione Vitae Humanae* (*On the Conservation of Human Life*, c.1307-08), affirmed that it started as thirty-five. Jean Froissart's poem, *Le Joli Buisson de Jonece* (*The Fair Arbor of Youth*, 1373), wrote that old age commenced at fifty-eight. By taking the average age from the previous works, one can get an idea about when old age was thought to begin.[3]

It is difficult to know whether the authors of the preceding works referred to men and women or to men only. However, Vincent de Beauvais stated that old age began at fifty, when women could no longer have children: "The fourth stage of youth ceases in the fiftieth year when one fails to produce offspring."[4]

From the preceding works, it can be assumed that medieval writers believed that old age began around the age of fifty—about the same time women experience menopause. Several medieval works have stated that women reached menopause around the age of fifty. Post-menopause begins one year after a woman stops menstruating and lasts until her death.[5] In the medical book, *Causae et Curae* (*Causes and Cures*, 1150), Hildegard of Bingen wrote: "The menses cease in women from the fiftieth year and sometimes in certain ones from the sixtieth when the uterus begins to be enfolded and to contract, so that they are no longer able to conceive." Thomas de Cantimpré's encyclopedic work, *De Natura Rerum*, avowed: "A woman conceives clear up to the fiftieth year."[6] Gilbertus Anglicus' medical book, *Compendium Medicinae* (*Compendium of Medicine*, c.1230-40) affirmed: "The menses are withheld naturally below twelve and above fifty years."[7] Bartholomaeus Anglicus' book, *De Rerum Proprietatibus*, stated: "The retention of the menses was to be a matter of concern generally from the fourteenth up to the fiftieth year."[8] In the thirteenth century medical work, *Lilium Medicinae* (*Lily of Medicine*, 1283-1308), Bernard de Gordon believed that the usual ages for menstruation were between fourteen and fifty.[9] John of Gaddesden's popular work, *Rosa Medicinae* (*Rose of Medicine*, 1305-17) asserted: "The menses are withheld naturally until twelve or fourteen years and after fifty, although in some cases they cease earlier, at thirty-five, forty, or forty-five, according to the various natures of women."[10] Thus, most medical writers during the Middle Ages assumed that menopause began around the age of fifty.

Since post-menopause is the final stage of life that can cover many years of a woman's life—from old age to extreme old age to death, I use the terms post-menopause, old, and elderly interchangeably throughout this book.

The main problem in reading medieval literature for a historical study is the scarcity of sources. Before the invention of the printing press (about 1450), books were a rarity. My sources consist of didactic and prescriptive works, literature, and evidence of lived lives. Many of my sources have been translated from Latin and French into English, which may pose some problems in its interpretation. Throughout the centuries, medieval texts have been translated and/or transcribed many times. Some of a source's original meaning could have been lost in the translation process. Through translation, some of the words, phrases, and/or sentences from the original texts could have been slightly or considerably altered, thus changing the original meaning. Moreover, several books from the medieval period, including manuscripts, have disappeared, been destroyed, or are missing sections. Manuscripts and books that were produced during the Middle Ages were hand copied by scribes and copiers. However, a scribe copying a book could have misinterpreted or misspelled a word, hence changing its original meaning. Since books were rare and expensive, only the wealthy could afford them.

Literacy was prevalent amongst the clergy, men of the middle and upper classes, nuns, and upper-class women. Medieval writers were chiefly men; only a few women were writers. This fact may have affected literary attitudes and perceptions toward women in general. Furthermore, the authorship of some medieval sources is either unknown or attributed to a number of authors.

The book is divided into four categories: historical context, didactic and prescriptive works, literature, and evidence of lived lives. Chapter 1, "A Time of Change for Women: 1100-1400 in Context," examines major events that affected the lives of women in Western Europe from 1100-1400. Chapter 2, "Didactic and Prescriptive Works on Old Age," analyzes the works of philosophers, medical, and religious writers in relation to the aging process, old age, and post-menopausal women. Chapter 3, "Old Women in Literature," investigates attitudes toward old women in poems, plays, and literature. Chapter 4, "The Lives of Post-Menopausal Women in the High and Late Middle Ages," looks at evidence of how post-menopausal women lived their lives in Western Europe during the High and Late Middle Ages. It examines the lives of abbesses, noble women, peasant women, and widows.

CHAPTER 1

A TIME OF CHANGE FOR WOMEN: 1100-1400 IN CONTEXT

The period of 1100-1400 witnessed several changes that affected the lives of women in Western Europe. The chapter looks at the development of heretical sects, such as the Cathars and the Béguines in the twelfth century and the Church's response to heresy in the subsequent centuries. The chapter further examines one of the most devastating plagues in history that produced massive demographic and economic changes in fourteenth-century Europe. The Black Death, along with the rise of commercialism and capitalism, brought economic changes that altered women's work roles in the post-plague years.

Heretical Religions

The twelfth century marked the emergence of the heretical religion known as Catharism. The precise year when the Cathars first appeared is unknown, but in 1163, they were first introduced in Eckbert of Schoenau's book, *13 Sermons against the Cathars*. The Cathars originated in the Low Countries and Germany and spread to the south of France. The Cathars were also known as the Albigensians for their prevalence in the southern French town of Albi.[11]

The Cathar movement attracted female converts from all social strata. The Cathars included nobles and peasants, young girls and old women, women separated from their husbands, and widows. Cathar women came from such noble French families as de Puylaurens, Laurac, Mirot, and

Mirepoix. During the twelfth and early thirteenth centuries, some Cathar noble women set up female religious houses in southern France, where they had workshops, clinics, and schools.[12] The historian, Emmanuel Le Roy Ladurie noted the presence of several elderly Cathar woman in the early fourteenth-century French peasant village of Montaillou (see chapter 4).

The Cathars defied everything that the Catholic Church stood for. They rivaled the Church's hierarchies by forming their own Cathar bishops, dioceses, councils, and popes. Instead of practicing a monotheistic religion like Christianity, the Cathars believed in a dualistic religion consisting of two deities, one of good (God) and the other of evil (Satan). They further held that evil forces created the body, while good forces produced the soul. The Cathars denied purgatory, masses for the dead, transubstantiation, and infant baptism. Cathar marriage was not a sacrament and divorce was allowed.[13]

The main religious ceremony was known as the consolamentum, where the believer was freed from his or her physical body and reunited with his or her pure and sinless spirit. This event mostly took place at the time of death and was administered by the spiritual elite called Perfecti or Perfects. Both, Cathar men and women became Perfects. The Perfects practiced chastity, owned no property, ate no meat, and lived in complete austerity. Female Perfects could preach and administer the consolamentum to women and to men, if the male Perfect was absent. In the Cathar religion, female Perfects were able to perform certain religious functions that were barred to Catholic laywomen and women in approved religious orders.[14]

For instance, in 1210, Pope Innocent III issued a papal bull *Nova Quaedam Nuper*, in which he criticized abbesses who "bless their nuns, hear their confessions of sins, and reading the gospel, presume to preach publicly."[15] He instructed bishops to stop abbesses from performing these services because "although the blessed Virgin Mary was worthier and more excellent than all the apostles, still the Lord commended the keys of the kingdom of heaven not to her, but to them [the apostles]."[16] In 1215, the Fourth Lateran Council barred women in religious orders and laypeople from preaching and hearing confessions. Under canons three, ten, and twenty-one of the Fourth Lateran Council, only priests could hear confessions, while preaching was limited to members of the clergy (bishops, priests, deacons).[17]

In 1204, at the age of about fifty-two, Countess Esclarmonde of Foix (c.1152-1215), sister of the count of Foix, widow of a lord in Gascony, and head of a Cathar convent in Pamiers, became a Perfect and frequently took part in debates between Cathars and Catholics. According to the chronicler

Guillaume de Puylaurens, Esclarmonde infuriated one Catholic cleric so much during a debate at Pamiers in 1207 that he stated: "Madame, go home and spin threads. It is not meet [proper] for a woman to take part in a religious discussion!"[18] As a female Perfect, Esclarmonde challenged Church authority and its hierarchy by participating in a heretical sect and taking part in religious discussions.

Around the mid-twelfth century, the Church began to persecute the Cathars. In 1163, the Council of Tours under Pope Alexander III required the clergy to inquire into heretical sects and to imprison and confiscate the property of anyone involved in these sects. At the Council of Verona (1184), Pope Lucius III issued the bull *Ad Abolendam* that condemned the Cathars as well as other heretical groups, prohibited anyone from preaching without papal permission, and denounced those who aided heretics. Bishops were to investigate parishes for heretics and anyone who acted suspiciously. Those convicted were excommunicated and punished by the secular authorities.[19]

However, these measures proved ineffective against heresy. More than twenty-five years later, Innocent III, in 1204, chose the Cistercian Abbot of Cîteaux, Arnaud-Amaury, and two monks, Peter of Castelnau and Ralph of Fontfroide, to lead a preaching mission in Languedoc, where Catharism was prevalent. Their preaching mission failed, the Cathars remained unyielding, and Peter of Castelnau was assassinated. In 1208, Pope Innocent III launched the Albigensian Crusade (1209-29) and placed Arnaud-Amaury in command. Arnaud-Amaury and his army plundered, burned, and massacred the population of Béziers in 1209. The Albigensian Crusade continued in a series of sieges for many years.[20]

In 1233, Pope Gregory IX, aided by the Dominicans and the Franciscans, embarked on an Inquisition against Catharism. It became the duty of the Dominicans and the Franciscans to determine the guilt or innocence of the accused by asking a series of questions, and if guilty, persuading them to recant. If proven guilty, offenders were punished by the secular authorities—usually by being imprisoned or burned. Those who repented had to do penance and wear a yellow cross on their clothing. In 1252, the Inquisition was allowed to employ torture. Between the Albigensian Crusade and the Inquisition, Catharism began to die out. By 1275, there was no French Cathar bishop left in France and in 1326, the last known French Cathar was burned at Carcassonne.[21]

Another heretical sect that evolved around the same time as the Cathars was the Béguines. The Béguine movement emerged in the Low Countries,

Germany, and France in the late twelfth and early thirteenth centuries. Why did the Béguine movement appear during this period? Jeffrey Richards suggests that the growth of mysticism in the Low Countries and Germany in the later Middle Ages contributed to one's discontentment with the existing forms of religious life. Marcia Guttentag and Paul F. Secord propose that there was a low sex ratio resulting from the increasing life expectancy of women during this period and therefore, a surplus of women. According to Guttentag and Secord, convents were too exclusive and too few in number to admit a large number of women. Shulamith Shahar added that many poor women joined the Béguines because they were unable to pay the required entrance fee to enter a convent.[22]

Women from every stage in life joined the Béguines, and this movement included young girls, old women, married women who had separated from their husbands, unmarried women, and widows.[23] The Béguines sought a less isolated religious life that would provide greater contact with other people in the community. They formed religious houses and lived together in communities called Béguinages where they worked and lived like Christ. They lived a life of poverty, aided the poor and the sick, did manual labor, practiced chastity, provided education to the young, preached, begged, and sought a personal relationship with God. Unlike nuns, the Béguines did not take a lifetime vow or belong to an institutionalized religious order. They did not follow a common rule, a general supervisory system, or a standard hierarchy and were allowed to leave the Béguinage at any time.[24]

As the Béguine movement expanded in size and popularity throughout the Low Countries, Germany, and France during the thirteenth and early fourteenth centuries, the Church grew ever more wary of the Béguines. The Church was distressed with the idea of women living in independent religious communities outside the boundaries of Church authority. Moreover, the Church was angry with some of the Béguines for interpreting and translating the Bible into German and French, which was forbidden by the Church. The Church believed that these tasks should be executed by clerics only. Some Béguines were denounced as heretics, such as the sixty-year-old Marguerite Porète of Hainaut (c.1250-1310), who on 1 June 1310 was burned at the stake in Paris by inquisitors for refusing to recant her heretical work on mysticism entitled, *Le Mirouer des Simples Ames* (*The Mirror of Simple Souls*).[25]

In the early 1300s, Pope Clement V issued a set of decrees called the Clementine decrees, which described the Béguines as an "abominable sect of women" who misled the faithful with their "wrong" beliefs and as "foolish women who have gotten into matters far too complicated for them to handle and who, as a result, are causing much confusion and trouble."[26] He further viewed them as "uneducated women who were confusing themselves and others by their unlawful preaching." Consequently, Clement V condemned their way of life, prohibited religious advisors from helping them, and issued housing restrictions that would move them off the streets and out of individual houses and into communities where they could be better supervised and controlled.[27]

At the Council of Vienne (1311-12), Pope Clement V released a papal bull that officially eradicated the Béguines since they violated the 1215 and 1274 bans on forming new orders. The 1215 Fourth Lateran Council and the 1274 Second Council of Lyons prohibited the formation of any new order and declared that every new religious community had to be within the rule of an accepted order.[28] The Council of Vienne further condemned the Béguines for their heretical beliefs. One of the Vienne decrees, *Cum de Quibusdam Mulieribus*, stated that some of the Béguines "discussed and preached about the Trinity and divine essence and expressed opinions contrary to the Catholic faith as if driven by a particular insanity."[29] To enforce the decrees and root out heresy, the Council of Vienne ordered bishops to conduct inquiries and monitor the behavior of suspect Béguines. Bishops were to convict suspect Béguines of heresy if they were found guilty. In 1320, Béguines who caused trouble were expelled from St. Christophe in Liège. Between 1320-21, the bishops of the dioceses of Thérouanne, Arras, Cambrai, Tournai, and Liège performed inquiries on Béguine communities.[30]

The persecuting decrees issued by Pope Clement V (the Clementine and Vienne decrees) may have contributed to the significant decline of Béguinages founded during the fourteenth century and in the following centuries. In Walter Simons' study of 298 Béguinages in 111 towns and cities in the southern Low Countries between 1200-1565, he discovered that the number of Béguinages established decreased as the decades progressed. The most dramatic drop in the number of Béguinages established during Simons' period of study (1200-1565) occurred between 1311-30—shortly after the Clementine and Vienne decrees. Thirty-four Béguinages were founded between 1311-20, but in the subsequent decade (1321-30), only eight were established. Furthermore, the largest drop in the number of Béguinages founded during the period of Simons' analysis took place in the fourteenth century. There were 205 Béguinages founded in the Southern Low Countries between 1200-1320, seventy-four between 1321-1400, and thirty-six between 1401-1565. In addition to the diminishing number of Béguinages founded, over fifty Béguinages in the southern Low Countries were closed (or were dropped from the records) by 1350, while another thirty-five were shut down by the end of the fourteenth century.[31]

The Black Death

Around the same time as Béguinages were fading from view, Europe was undergoing catastrophic demographic changes from the effects of the Black Death (1347-50). Within a few years, the plague wiped out more than a third of Europe's population. The plague, as well as other epidemics, tended to primarily target children and young adults while sparing the elderly. The English chronicler, Geoffrey le Baker, whose account spanned the period from 1303 to 1356, described the plague in 1349 England as besetting the young, while evading the old: "This disaster [plague] chiefly overwhelmed the young and strong; the elderly and weak it generally spared."[32] In 1383, the Italian chronicler Marchionne Stefani commented: "Many good people died, but the plague killed more young people and children than mature men and women."[33] Why did the plague kill the young and spare the old? The demographer Josiah C. Russell provided the following explanation:

> After the first plague epidemic, the children were particularly vulnerable to further outbreaks as they had been less exposed, or not exposed at all, beforehand.[34]

Children and young adults were more susceptible to the plague and other diseases because they had not built up enough immunity to ward them off. For instance, after the plague, tuberculosis largely killed those between the ages of fifteen and thirty-five. Those who survived childhood and young adulthood had a better chance of reaching old age. In fact, after the Black Death, there was a gradual rise in the life expectancy of the elderly while there was a sharp decline in the life expectancy of the younger generations. T. H. Hollingsworth's and J. C. Russell's demographic study on 3,070 English landowners throughout the Late Middle Ages illustrated:

> The average life expectancy at birth, which had been 35.3 years for men born between 1200 and 1275, had already decreased to 27.2 years for those men born between 1326 and 1348, falling to

17.3 years for the generation born in 1348-75 before gradually increasing to 32.8 years for the 1425-50 generation. On the other hand, the life expectancy of 60-year-old men climbed from 9.4 years for those born between 1200 and 1275 to 10.8 years for those born between 1326 and 1348, 10.9 years for the 1348-75 generation and 13.7 years for the 1425-50 generation. The life expectancy of 80-year-old men in the same periods climbed from 5.2 years to 6 years, 4.7 years and 7.9 years respectively.[35]

It would take a hundred years for the average life expectancy of men to exceed its pre-plague figures (1326-48). Yet, the average life expectancy of men born between 1425-50 did not equal or surpass the average life expectancy of men born between 1200 and 1275.

In a demographic study of medieval England, Josiah C. Russell discovered that the elderly population grew as the centuries progressed. Russell collected his data from inquisitions post mortem. After a landowner's death, the courts conducted inquisitions in regards to his landholdings. In addition, the inquisitions provided details on the names and ages of the landowners' heirs. He then compiled the age of inheritance and the age of death of 3,400 individuals. From this data, Russell observed that the elderly made up 6.9 percent of the adult population in England between 1301-25, 8.9 percent between 1326-48, 10.3 percent between 1348-75, 9.0 percent between 1376-1400, 10.6 percent between 1401-25. Hence, the elderly population in England continued to rise before, during, and after the Black Death. Though the elderly population slightly declined between 1376-1400, its percentage soon exceeded its previous figures between 1401-25.[36]

Joel T. Rosenthal's study of the longevity of the English peerage during the fourteenth century showed that the mortality rate increased for those under fifty, while the mortality rate decreased for those over fifty:

> Before 1325 18 percent of peers died before they reached the age of 50; the ratio increased to 66 percent between 1350 and 1370 before decreasing to 34 percent during the first half of the fifteenth century. However those who did turn 50 lived much longer.[37]

Since Hollingsworth's and Russell's statistics applied only to men, could their statistics apply to women as well? Maybe so. The life expectancy of women increased during the High Middle Ages and steadily surpassed the life expectancy of men. The rise in the life expectancy of women was partially due to the increase intake of iron and protein in the medieval diet. Women increased their protein and iron intake by practicing new farming techniques, using iron pots, and by consuming more meat and protein-rich legumes. The increase intake of iron was beneficial to women who required it for the loss of blood during menstruation, pregnancy, and childbirth and almost certainly reduced anemia-related deaths in women. Moreover, J. C. Russell's analysis on the skeletal remains of elderly males and females during the plague period (1348-1500) demonstrated that females were almost as numerous as males. The study was conducted in over five hundred cemeteries in mainly northern and eastern Europe. The skeletal remains showed that there were 3.3 percent males and 3.2 percent females.[38] In addition, the increasing life expectancy of women was commented on by the late thirteenth century biologist and writer, Albertus Magnus. Albertus somewhat overturned Aristotle's and Vincent de Beauvais' views on males living longer than females. Both, Aristotle's *On the Length and Shortness of Life* and Vincent de Beauvais' work, *Speculum Naturale*, professed that men lived longer than women since males were warmer than females. However, Albertus Magnus wrote that "men by nature live longer than women, for the reason that they were warmer, but per accidens [by accident] women in fact live longer than men" since "they [women] work less, and are not so much consumed."[39]

The Black Death caused major demographic changes in Europe. It killed off the young in great numbers while sparing the old and increasing their longevity. Even though the plague killed off more than a third of Europe's population, the elderly population continued to grow throughout the plague and post-plague period.

Women and Work

The economic condition of post-plague England significantly affected women's work and status. Patriarchy, capitalism, commercialism, and a series of regulations sought to limit or exclude women from the commercial sphere in post-plague England. One group that was affected by the economic situation of post-plague England were female ale brewers (also known as brewsters), especially those who were single or widowed. In Judith M. Bennett's case study of brewsters in England between 1300-1600, she found that there was a dramatic decline in the number of unmarried and widowed brewsters after the plague. She believed that the commercialization and the capitalization of brewing, along with its increasing regulations, led to their decline.[40]

Before the Black Death, brewing was dominated by women in England since it was a domestic activity that brought little profit, investment, or entrepreneurial interest. Women brewed ale for their families' consumption and sold it to supplement their husbands' incomes. In pre-plague Brigstock, Northamptonshire, one-third of the women (more than 300 women) on the manor brewed ale. In Wakefield, Yorkshire, between 1348 and 1350 one-third of the women (185 women) brewed ale. There were more married brewsters than single or widowed brewsters since most adult women were married. In an court roll from Wallingford in 1228-29, eighty percent of brewsters were married. In early fourteenth-century Tamworth, two-thirds of brewsters were married. In 1311, in Oxford, twenty-eight brewsters were single or widowed, while one hundred and nine were married. In 1348, in Oxford, fourteen brewsters were single or widowed, while seventy-four were married. Although single and widowed brewsters were always a minority, their numbers grew less and less after the plague.[41]

Before the Black Death, few men identified themselves as brewers. Male brewers usually worked alongside their wives or less frequently on their own. Of the thousands of men who entered their occupations to the freedom of York before the plague, only one man, Alan de Munkton, claimed to be a brewer in 1336-37.[42]

However, as brewing expanded and became more profitable after the Black Death, more men became brewers. Between 1350-99, seven men entered the freedom of York as brewers and dozens more followed suit during the fifteenth century. Furthermore, in Kibworth Harcourt, Leicestershire, husbands of brewsters were cited more frequently in court during the 1350s and 1360s, as more males became servants in brewing households. In late fourteenth-century Oxford, brewers hired three male servants for every two female servants.[43]

As the centuries progressed, ale brewing became increasingly regulated, especially after the plague. Before the thirteenth century, England regulated ale by levying a toll on commercial brewing called a tolcester. By the thirteenth century, local authorities began using tighter controls on commercial brewing with the assize of ale. The assize of ale was a statute that regulated the price of ale. Local officers called aletasters supervised commercial brewers and enforced the assize of ale statute. If brewers disobeyed the statute then they went to court. Brewers were subject to fines if they sold ale in dishonest measures, ale of poor quality, or at extreme prices. By the fourteenth century, commercial brewers all over England were expected to observe the assize of ale. After 1350, communities began to supervise brewers more directly and called for all brewers to publicize their ale. Although brewing was predominantly a female occupation, those who regulated the ale trade—aletasters, bailiffs, juries, and mayors were all men.[44]

After the plague, significant changes took place in the English ale trade. Ale grew in popularity after the plague as milk and cider decreased in popularity. With a rise in wages and an overall higher standard of living, people (especially among the working classes in urban and rural areas) consumed more ale per capita than before. As ale grew in popularity and profits, brewing became an industrial and commercial enterprise. It changed low-profit cottage industry to a high-profit profession. Commercial brewing moved from private households to public brewhouses.[45]

As brewing expanded and became more commercialized after the plague, it required more capital, skill, equipment, and assistance than before. Those who had money to invest in the ale trade had an advantage over smaller brewers since they owned larger premises for brewing, could hire more workers, and possessed better brewing equipment. Moreover, brewers sometimes needed to take out loans in order to finance their businesses.[46]

The expansion and commercialization of the ale trade disadvantaged women, particularly unmarried women and widows. It was difficult for unmarried women and widows to obtain cash and credit because they were viewed as poor credit risks. In general, women owned less property and earned lower wages than men. Consequently, they were not considered dependable debtors. Since married women could not sign contracts, their husbands could take out loans for them. Even though single and widowed women could independently make contracts and contract loans, they usually borrowed less than married women. In Maryanne Kowaleski's analysis of debt cases from 1378-88 Exeter, Devonshire, the average debt of single women was 4s. 6d., 10s. 1d. for wives, who appeared in the debt case with their husbands, and 14s. for men. From Kowaleski's study, women tended to borrow from other women, acquired smaller loans than men (one-third to one-half less), and borrowed money for domestic uses rather than for business uses.[47]

With limited access to cash and credit to expand their trade, unmarried and widowed brewsters decreased in numbers. In the court records of Stockton, Wiltshire, unmarried and widowed brewsters comprised of twenty percent between 1281-99, thirteen percent between 1306-44, and eleven percent between 1349-99. In Norwich, there were sixteen percent of unmarried and widowed brewsters in 1288 and seven percent in 1390. On the manor of Cranborne, Dorset, twenty-nine percent of unmarried and widowed women were in court for ale violations in 1330, but only three percent appeared before the court in 1380. On the manor of Preston-on-Wye, Herefordshire, fourteen percent of unmarried and widowed women were in court for ale infractions in 1275, thirty-three percent in 1320, and a combined nine percent for 1366 and 1395.[48]

As brewsters, single women and widows enjoyed a slightly higher standard of living than other unmarried women in other professions. Although they were not as prosperous as single men or married couples in the ale trade, single and widowed brewsters participated in a reasonably skilled profession that brought some affluence. For instance, in 1379, the town of Howden, England, consisted of nine unmarried and widowed brewsters, eleven married brewsters, and one male brewer. Most of the unmarried and widowed women in Howden worked in unskilled jobs as servants and laborers and paid the minimum of 4d. in poll tax. In contrast, the nine unmarried and widowed brewsters in Howden paid 6d. to 12d. in poll tax.[49]

As brewing became more profitable after the Black Death, unmarried and widowed brewsters were marginalized in the least lucrative positions of the ale trade. From the Oxford Assizes, we learn that there were twenty-eight female-headed households in 1311 where the heads worked as brewsters, while twenty-six female heads of households worked in the less lucrative position of tippling (selling ale, not brewing it). In 1351, five female heads of households brewed ale, while sixteen female heads of households sold ale. In the poll tax of 1381, twenty-nine households brewed ale in Oxford. Of the twenty-nine households, only five households were headed by unmarried or widowed female brewsters, twelve sold ale, and eighteen worked as servants in brewing households. At the close of the fourteenth century, the number of single and widowed brewsters declined as the ale trade expanded into the commercial realm.[50]

The period of 1100-1400 affected the lives of European women in several ways. It was a period of decline in power and status for women that coincided with the rise of Church power. To root out heresy and to maintain its authority, the Church persecuted heretical sects, such as the Cathars and the Béguines. The Church issued decrees, launched a Crusade and an Inquisition against these groups until they disappeared or were drastically reduced in numbers. The period of the Black Death produced distressing effects on demographics. The plague killed off the young in large numbers while sparing the elderly population and increasing their longevity. The post-plague economy, along with the growth of capitalism and commercialism, sought to restrict or exclude women, such as brewsters, from participating in the commercial sphere. These events impacted the lives of women in work, religion, and society.

CHAPTER 2

DIDACTIC AND PRESCRIPTIVE WORKS ON OLD AGE

Didactic and prescriptive writers in the High and Late Middle Ages held diverse views on the topic of old age. The chapter analyzes some of these views in relation to the aging process and the aged, second childhoods, and post-menopausal women. In regard to aging, Hildegard of Bingen perceived the aging process as a natural part of life, while Roger Bacon viewed it as a time of physical and mental decline. Bartholomaeus Anglicus and Philip de Novare associated old age with childhood since they shared similar mental characteristics. Other medieval writers focused on post-menopausal women in regard to their inability to love, their deviant ways, and their harmful bodies. Andreas Capellanus thought that women lost their capability to love at the age of fifty and Philip de Novare criticized post-menopausal women for not acting their age. Moreover, Albertus Magnus believed that menopausal and post-menopausal women were venomous and dangerous to children.

The Aging Process and The Aged

In Hildegard of Bingen's three-part work of religious history, Church doctrine, and visions entitled, *Scivias* (*Know the Ways*, 1141-51), she viewed old age as a natural occurrence in life. Ten complete manuscripts of *Scivias* exist, six of them are dated from the twelfth century. In *Scivias I*, Hildegard wrote:

The soul reveals her capabilities according to the capabilities of
the body, so that in childhood she brings forth simplicity, in
youth strength, and in the fullness of age, when all the veins of
the human being are full, she brings forth her greatest strength
in wisdom. In the same way a tree in its first growth brings forth
tender shoots, goes on then to bear fruit and finally ripens that
fruit to the fullness of utility. But afterwards in old age when a
human being's bones and veins incline to weakness, then the soul
reveals gentler strengths, as though tired of human knowledge.
In the same way, at the onset of wintertime, the sap of the tree
withdraws from the leaves and branches as the tree begins to
incline towards old age.[51]

Hildegard's passage regarding the life stages was intended for women
since she was describing the female soul. She associated old age with the
changing of the seasons. Like the seasons, human beings go through a
continuous cycle of birth, life, and death. Although Hildegard correlated
old age with frailty, she still portrayed the aging process with respect when
she stated: "the soul reveals gentler strengths."[52] Instead of using the word
weakness to describe the soul, Hildegard chose to utilize the word strength.
Her positive tone towards old age could have been a reflection of her own
active and spiritual life.

In the philosophical work entitled, *Opus Majus* (*Greater Work*, c.1266),
the English philosopher, Roger Bacon took a negative stance on old age.
Opus Majus was a well-known work in its time. In 1266, Pope Clement IV
wrote a letter to Bacon asking him to send copies of his works. Accordingly,
Bacon sent *Opus Majus* to the pope.[53]

In *Opus Majus*, Roger Bacon believed that the prime of life ended
around the age of forty-five or fifty. He described the prime of life as being
"the age of human beauty and strength," which preceded old age and
senility.[54] Bacon explained old age as follows:

All these accidents of old age and senility are white hair, pallor,
wrinkling of the skin, excess of mucus, foul phlegm, inflammation
of the eyes, and general injury to the organs of sense, diminution
of blood and of the spirits, weakness in motion and breathing
and in the whole body, failure in both the animal and natural
powers of the soul, sleeplessness, anger and disquietude of the
mind and forgetfulness.[55]

To Bacon, old age consisted of mental and physical decrepitude. He employed a series of negative words, such as accidents, senility, foul, injury, diminution, weakness, and failure to depict the characteristics of old age. In regard to old age, Roger Bacon mentioned the Arab physician, Hali Ibn Abbas and the Greek philosopher, Plato.[56] Bacon noted: "The royal Hali says that old age is the home of forgetfulness; and Plato that it is the mother of lethargy."[57]

Second Childhood

Since old age was characterized as the weakening of the mind and body, the idea of a second childhood emerged. It was thought by some that older people reverted to childhood. Although the notion of a second childhood was not exclusive to the Middle Ages, it was a common theme in medieval writings.[58]

Bartholomaeus Anglicus' enormously well-known scientific encyclopedia, *De Rerum Proprietatibus* (c.1230-40) associated the elderly with children in terms of their character. Bartholomaeus Anglicus was an English Franciscan monk whose work served as a reference book for his fellow Franciscans. In addition, this work gained mass wide appeal. From the late thirteenth century to the sixteenth century, *De Rerum Proprietatibus* was translated from Latin into English, French, Provençal, Italian, Spanish, German, and Dutch. In 1297, Pope Boniface VIII donated the book to a Dominican convent.[59]

In *De Rerum Proprietatibus*, Bartholomaeus Anglicus perceived children and old people as having comparable traits since they both shared similar humors. Bartholomaeus wrote:

> Those who have cold blood are foolish and those who have warm blood are wise and have great prudence in their nature . . . and for this old people whose blood is cooled, and children whose blood is not yet warmed up are not wise like others.[60]

Bartholomaeus Anglicus distinguished childhood and old age from the other life stages because they shared similar qualities. Therefore, he deemed children and old people foolish and lacking in judgment because they, unlike those between childhood and old age, possessed cold blood.

Philip de Novare was an Italian soldier, historian, lawyer, and diplomat who wrote a didactic work on the human life cycle entitled, *Les Quatre Ages de l'Homme* (c1260). The work exists in five manuscripts dating from the thirteenth and fifteenth centuries.[61] In it, Philip de Novare associated the middle-aged mindset to that of children. He wrote:

> The "middle aged" have lost much of their worth and knowledge, they are forgetful and confused and have entered their second childhood and merit only the respect due to children.[62]

According to Philip de Novare, those who were middle-aged were between the ages of forty and sixty, while those who were old were between the ages of sixty and eighty. He noted that there were a few who lived to be eighty, but they should pray for death since their lives were so miserable.[63] According to Philip, from the age of forty on, one became absentminded, insignificant, and undignified. Hence, the middle-aged entered into their second childhoods once their mental capabilities (intellect, knowledge, memory) began to falter. The middle-aged were to be treated like children since their mental functions were on par with those of children. Like children, the middle-aged were no longer able to work and became financially dependent on others.

Post-Menopausal Women

In the works of Andreas Capellanus and Philip de Novare, post-menopausal women were subjected to a strict code of conduct in regard to love and sex. They were to behave appropriately to their age. After reaching an age that was conventionally accepted as marking the end of fertility, women were to cease sexual activity, and forgo desire and lead celibate lives. Love and sex were meant for the young, not for the old. Those who remained sexually active were condemned and ridiculed by medieval writers.

Andreas Capellanus' work, *The Art of Courtly Love* (c.1184-86) asserted that post-menopausal women were incapable of romantic love. Not much is known about Andreas Capellanus, but he was most likely a chaplain for the French court. He wrote *The Art of Courtly Love* at the request of Countess Marie of Champagne and Troyes, daughter of Eleanor of Aquitaine and Louis VII of France.[64]

The Art of Courtly Love was a popular advice manual on love. Twelve manuscripts of *The Art of Courtly Love* exist. Andreas Capellanus' work was translated into Italian, German, French, and Catalan.[65]

According to Andreas Capellanus, love disappeared for women at the age of fifty and for men at the age of sixty. He explained:

> Age is a bar, because after the sixtieth year in a man and the fiftieth in a woman, although one may have intercourse his passion cannot develop into love; because at that age the natural heat begins to lose its force, and the natural moisture is greatly increased, which leads a man into various difficulties and troubles him with various ailments.[66]

Andreas Capellanus provided a reason why love disappeared for men, but not for women. He mentioned the age at which women lost their ability to love, but he did not provide an explanation. However, it can be assumed from the specific age Andreas chose (50 years), that love disappeared for women around menopause.[67]

Philip de Novare believed that post-menopausal women should accept the fact that they are old and undesirable. In his didactic work, *Les Quatre Ages de l'Homme*, Philip de Novare advised older women to start acting their age since nothing was more ridiculous than a woman past her reproductive years trying to behave like a young woman. To Philip, old women should set a moral example for the young by helping the poor, doing penance, praying, fasting, taking care of children, managing the household, and arranging marriages. Conversely, post-menopausal women who wore make-up, dyed their hair, dressed in fine clothes, and remained sexually active were viewed by Philip de Novare as evil, foolish, pathetic, and in denial. According to Philip, post-menopausal women remained sexually active because they were afraid to admit that they were old and finished. These women were so desperate to satisfy their vanity they paid men to have sex with them. To him, a woman past childbearing age stopped having sex because no man wanted her. Therefore, Philip de Novare believed that post-menopausal women were sexually useless and undesirable to men.[68]

The restrictions placed on a post-menopausal woman's sexuality was partially due to the Christian notion that the sole purpose of sex was for procreation. Having sex for any other reason was deemed unnatural and immoral. The highly influential theologian, St. Augustine believed that sex was a necessary evil for the continuation of humankind. For him, celibacy was the highest virtue. Reminiscent of St. Augustine, the thirteenth century theologians St. Albertus Magnus and St. Thomas Aquinas considered virginity and celibacy more virtuous than sexual activity. The medieval church looked upon sex during old age as a sin against nature since it did not lead to procreation. Those who defied religious teaching and remained sexually active in their old age were viewed by the church as lustful and deviant. Therefore, according to the Church, sexual activity was allowed to women only during their reproductive years. Once a woman reached menopause, she was to abstain from sexual activity and lead a virtuous, celibate existence.[69]

An old woman's body was sometimes depicted in medieval writings as dangerous, venomous, and contagious to children. In the late thirteenth century medical and philosophical treatise, *De Secretis Mulierum* (*Women's Secrets*), by German philosopher, scientist, and theologian Albertus Magnus, old women had the power to infect and kill children. It was a well-known and extremely popular work in Europe. Over fifty editions of *De Secretis Mulierum* were printed in the fifteenth century and over seventy editions were printed in the sixteenth century.[70]

Albertus Magnus regarded menopausal and post-menopausal women as more dangerous than menstruating women. He stated: "The retention of menses engenders many evil humours. The women being old have almost no natural heat to consume and control this matter."[71] In his conception of the female body, menstruating women could purge venomous humors from their bodies while non-menstruating women retained them within their bodies. Since menopausal and post-menopausal women did not possess enough natural heat to expel these humors, they became even more poisonous than menstruating women.[72]

Albertus Magnus further believed that the humors of old women and poor women were more poisonous than the humors of other women since the poor ate coarse food and the old did not work. Women who were old and/or poor were more likely to infect and kill children with their eyes since they were extremely poisonous. This polluted air infected and killed children. Albertus claimed that old women poisoned the eyes of children by simply glancing at them. He advised old women not to play with children or kiss them because they could poison and kill them. Children were more easily infected by venomous humors because their bodies were more sensitive and porous than those of adults. However, women did not poison themselves because their bodies were accustomed to possessing and expelling venomous substances, such as menstrual blood.[73]

The notion of evil humors escaping through the eyes of women was mentioned in Aristotle's *On Animals*. According to Aristotle, the humors leave the body through the eyes because the eyes are watery. Therefore, women cry a lot because they have too much moisture in their bodies and crying rids the excess moisture.[74]

The idea of menstrual blood being impure was not a new concept in the Middle Ages. However, it was not until the thirteenth century that this concept was regularly addressed in European academic scientific treatises. With the rise of universities and Latin translations of classical works from the Arabic world, medieval scientific writers in the twelfth and thirteenth centuries rediscovered the writings of the ancient Greeks and Romans.[75]

Didactic and prescriptive writers in the High and Late Middle Ages held mostly negative attitudes toward aging and the aged, especially old women. Apart from the optimistic views of Hildegard of Bingen toward old age, Roger Bacon, Philip de Novare, Bartholomaeus Anglicus, Andreas Capellanus, and Albertus Magnus perceived the aging process, old age, and post-menopausal women in a negative light. To Roger Bacon and Philip de Novare, growing older brought forgetfulness, weakness, less respect, and mental and physical anguish. Since old age was characterized with the weakening of the mind and body, authors, such as Bartholomaeus Anglicus and Philip de Novare compared old age with childhood. Old people, or in Philip de Novare's case, middle-aged people, were like children because they shared similar qualities. In the works of Albertus Magnus, Philip de Novare, and Andreas Capellanus, post-menopausal women were deemed dangerous, improper, and unable to love. They were ridiculed and criticized for not conforming to age-appropriate behavior if they remained sexually active and tried to look and act like young women. These views were not only expressed by didactic and prescriptive writers, but were shared by many literary writers as well. Medieval literature often ran parallel with didactic and prescriptive works in their attitudes toward old women.

CHAPTER 3

OLD WOMEN IN LITERATURE

Writers in the High and Late Middle Ages often depicted old women in poems, plays, and other literary works as lusty, spurned by love/ lover, as go-betweens, having extraordinary powers, poor, and useless. Geoffrey Chaucer and the anonymous French work, *Les Quinze Joies de Mariage* (*The Fifteen Joys of Marriage*, c.1390) portrayed old women as sexually assertive bawds who dominated over their (usually younger) husbands. Conon de Béthune and Jean de Meun wrote about old women who were spurned by love/lovers because they were no longer young and attractive. The anonymous Latin play, *Pamphilus* (c.1100-50) and Giovanni Boccaccio illustrated old women as impoverished go-betweens who arranged clandestine meetings between young lovers. In the works of John Gower and Geoffrey Chaucer, old women were depicted as having extraordinary powers. They had the power to transform themselves from repulsive old hags into beautiful young women. Other medieval writers, such as, Wolfram von Eschenbach, Chaucer, and Boccaccio described old women as either impoverished, useless, or limited in their abilities. The chapter examines some of the characterizations made by medieval writers concerning old women.

Lusty Old Women

Geoffrey Chaucer's immensely popular satirical work, *The Canterbury Tales* (c.1385-1400) portrayed a lusty and sexually manipulative character in the form of Alison, the Wife of Bath. This widely known work exists in eighty-two manuscripts dating from c.1400 to 1490.[76]

In Chaucer's "The Wife of Bath's Prologue," Alison described herself as a widow who had outlived five husbands and was looking for husband number six. As soon as one husband died, she would quickly marry another. She married in rapid succession because she did not want to lead a celibate existence.[77] Alison resisted the traditional notion that older widows should remain chaste. Even though she was an older widow, Alison was determined to find another husband and resume an active sex life.

As a wife, Alison enjoyed sex and having sexual mastery over her husbands:

> As a wife I'll use my instrument as generously as my Maker gave it. My husband shall have it night and morning whenever he wants to come and pay his dues. I shan't stop him! A husband I must have, one that is both my debtor and my slave; and so long as I'm his wife he'll have his "tribulation of the flesh". While I'm alive I'm given "the power of his own body" and not he.[78]

In turn, she refused to have sex with those who disobeyed her authority. Alison cunningly remarked:

> So I can boast of one thing: in the end I got the better of my husbands in every way, by force, cunning, or one means and another, such as keeping up an everlasting grumbling and natter. Especially in bed their luck was out; that's where I'd scold and do them out of their fun. When I felt my husband's arm come over my side I wouldn't stay another moment in the bed until he's ransomed himself to me; and then I'd let him do his foolishness.[79]

Alison married her first three husbands for money and the last two for love. She described her first three husbands as wealthy, old, and impotent. She considered the first three to be good husbands because they gave her the upper hand in marriage. They were so desperate to win her affections that they did not care if she bullied, scolded, and ridiculed them into submission. Alison expressed:

> The good three were rich and old, and could barely keep the contract that bound us—you know what I mean by that! So help me God it makes me laugh whenever I think how unmercifully

I made them work of nights! And I thought nothing of it, that I
swear! They'd given me their land and treasure, so I didn't need
to trouble myself further to win their love or show them respect.
Heaven's above, they loved me so much I set no value on it. But
as I had them in the hollow of my hand and had given me all
their lands already, why bother to please them except for my
profit and amusement? My word, I worked them hard—many's
the night I made them bawl! Yet I ruled them so well in my own
way that each was perfectly happy; they were always ready to
bring me pretty things from the fair. How glad they were when I
spoke to them nicely, for God knows how viciously I scolded.[80]

Clearly, Alison was a woman who knew about men. She used her
husbands for her own benefit. She pretended to love and respect them
in order to control their money and lands. Once she was given free rein
over their money and lands, she dropped the charade. Although Alison's
husbands loved her dearly and would do anything to make her happy, she
did not return their affection. Instead, she controlled her husbands and
treated them poorly. She was cruel in the sense that she took pleasure in
tormenting them and poking fun at their impotence. Still, they were happy
to be married to her.

In contrast to Alison's first three husbands, she married her last two
husbands for love. Even though she loved them, she considered them
bad husbands because they defied her authority. Her fourth husband was
unfaithful and kept a mistress while her fifth husband was domineering,
misogynistic, and physically abusive.[81]

In her fourth and fifth marriage, Alison assumed the same role as her
previous three husbands: older, rich, gullible, and desperate for affection.
When she married her fifth husband, she was forty and he was twenty. At
forty, Alison described herself as young and beautiful. Now, (she does not
mention her current age) she describes herself as old and ugly: "But age
alas! That cankers everything, has stripped me of my beauty and go."[82]

Similar to her previous husbands, Alison gave all of her money and
property (inherited from her past husbands) to her fifth husband, but
soon regretted it when he became too controlling. Though he physically
abused her, she continued to love him regardless. However, there were a
few instances when Alison attacked her husband for his misogynistic and
domineering ways. For instance, when her husband refused to stop reading
misogynistic literature from Greek, Roman, and biblical history, she hit

him in the face and tore three pages from his book. In retaliation, he hit her in the ear so hard that she went deaf in that one ear. After this incident, he promised never to hit her again and permitted her to rule over him, the house, the money, and the land. In the end, Alison gained mastery over her husband, but for a price.[83]

Alison of Bath ended her tale with the following statement:

> And may Jesus Christ send us husbands who are submissive, and young, and spirited in bed; and may He send us grace to outlive those we marry; and also I pray Jesus to shorten the days of those who'll not be governed by their wives; and as for old, bad-tempered, pennypinching skinflints, God's plague upon them![84]

Instead of the traditional idea of a husband ruling over his wife, Alison of Bath proposed that a wife should rule over her husband. She praised husbands who were young, vigorous, and obedient, while condemning those who were old, frugal, unkind, and defiant. By emphasizing supremacy in her own life and tale, Alison defended female sovereignty over male authority. Alison's idea of old women asserting power over men in relationships and in marriage during the Middle Ages challenged the traditional view of men having authority over women.

Like Chaucer, the anonymous French work, *Les Quinze Joies de Mariage* (c.1390) was a satirical work that advised young men against marrying old women since they are lusty, jealous, and possessive. Moreover, they cause distress and shorten their lifespan:

> There is no serf in greater bondage than a young, simple and carefree man who is subject to and ruled by a widow . . . he who falls into this state can do nothing beyond praying to God to give him patience to endure and suffer all . . . and it often happens, because he is very young compared with her, that she grows jealous: for her enjoyment and lechery with the young man and his young body makes her lustful and jealous, and she would like to have him in her arms at all times, and she would always like to be close. And indeed such old women married to young men are so jealous and so lustful that they are quite maddened and wherever the husband goes, whether to church or elsewhere, it seems to them it is only for wrongdoing. God knows what tribulation and torment he suffers and how he is assaulted. A

young woman would never be jealous for these reasons, and she would find a cure when she needed one. He who is in the situation I speak of is so brow-beaten that he dare not talk to any woman, and he must serve the lady who is old: because of which he will age more in a year than he would have done in ten years with a young wife. The old woman will squeeze him dry and he will live on in vexation and pain, in constant torment, and he will end his days miserably.[85]

The author of *Les Quinze Joies de Mariage* characterized young men as the helpless victims of female dominance and cruelty. They are governed by their much older wives and live a life of perpetual misery. In contrast to young women, old women are overbearing, jealous, and crave sex with young men in order to regain their lost youth: "She [the aged woman] finds a young man with a young body who renews her."[86] In turn, their constant jealousy and demands for sex will drain young men and thereby, shorten their lifespan. Within one year of marriage, a young man will age by ten years and if he remains with her, he will probably die an early death.

Throughout the Middle Ages, a marriage between an old woman and a young man could cause discord in the Church and in society. Given that religious dogma held that sex should be for reproductive purposes only, it was deemed unnatural for an old woman to marry a young man because their marriage would most likely be barren.[87] In his satirical poem, *Liber Lamentationum Matheoluli* (*The Lamentations of Matheolus*, c.1295), Mathieu of Boulogne warned men who wanted to get married to "try not to pick an old woman for they are sterile."[88]

Old Women Spurned by Love/Lover

The French trouvère, Conon de Béthune's lyric poem, "L'Autrier Avint en Chel Autre Païs" ("The Other Day It Happened in Another Land", c.1100-50) depicted an old woman who was spurned by her intended lover. He was a renowned poet of his time. Only ten of his lyric poems survive.[89]

Conon de Béthune's poem is a tale of a noble lady who refused a knight's love for a long time. When she finally fell in love with the knight, he turned her down because she was now old and ugly. The knight compared the lady's face to what he remembered:

The knight looked at her face, saw it very pale, its color gone. "Lady," he said, "it's my bad luck you didn't decide this long ago. Your bright face, that once looked like a lily, has gone, lady, from bad to worse, so that now I feel I have been robbed of you. Lady, you made up your mind too late."[90]

The knight's statement made the lady sound repulsive and unwanted. This led to a debate between the knight and the lady. She struck back at his harsh comments by stating that he was not good enough to love a great lady like herself. However, the knight argued that she lost her greatness a long time ago. To him, she was only beautiful in her youth. Although she was no longer young and beautiful, the lady believed that her wealth and noble status would attract men. She even mentioned a couple of men who still vied for her love. Nonetheless, the knight did not believe her and thought that the she was refusing to accept her age. He replied:

"Lady," he says, "it has bothered you very much that you have to rely on your high birth; but those seven who sighed for you in your youth, now, if you were the daughter of the king of Carthage, will not want to any more. One doesn't love a lady for her family, but when she is beautiful and courteous and wise. It won't be long before you learn the truth."[91]

According to the knight, once a woman reaches a certain age, she should forget about love since men admire youth and beauty, not old age and ugliness. Hence, the knight associated youth with beauty, good manners, and wisdom, and old age with ugliness, insolence, and foolishness. To him, physical beauty was more important than money and status.

The extremely popular French allegorical work, *Le Roman de la Rose* (*The Romance of the Rose*), included an old woman who was spurned by love and her lovers. It was written in two parts. Guillaume de Lorris wrote the first part between 1230-35 and Jean de Meun wrote the second part in 1275. *Le Roman de la Rose* enjoyed immense popularity from the thirteenth century until the sixteenth century when allegorical works fell out of fashion. Twenty-one editions of *Le Roman de la Rose* were printed between 1481 and 1538 and it was translated into Dutch, Italian, and English. One of the English translations is ascribed to Geoffrey Chaucer, who was fluent in French.[92]

In the second part of *Le Roman de la Rose* (1275), Jean de Meun portrayed La Vieille as a sexually deceptive character who was spurned by love and her lovers in her old age. La Vieille was a former prostitute who gave advice to a young man named Beu Accueil on the subject of sexual manipulation. La Vieille instructed Beu Accueil on this issue because she wanted him to learn from her mistakes. Furthermore, she wanted to protect him from being deceived by those who had once deceived her. La Vieille avowed:

> I want to teach you of the games of Love so that when you have learned them you will not be deceived. I was deceived by many before I noticed. Then it was too late, and I was miserably unhappy. I was already past my youth. I have no other way to avenge myself than by teaching my doctrine. Therefore, fair son, I indoctrinate you so that when instructed, you will avenge me on those good-for-nothings.[93]

By informing the younger generations about sexual exploitation and trickery, la Vieille sought vengeance on those who had cheated her. Therefore, she taught him how to manipulate men for money and gifts. She advised him to keep his heart in many places, not just one. In other words, Beu Accueil would receive more money and gifts if he took on several lovers instead of one. Moreover, she told him to never lend or give his heart away, but to always sell it to the "highest bidder". Thus, he should prey on men who are rich, gullible, and generous, while avoiding those who are poor, unkind, or miserly. To attract men, she advised him to decorate his clothes with fake jewels in order to appear more valuable. In addition, he should only give small, inexpensive gifts to those who would give better gifts in return. However, the most important word of advice la Vieille offered to Beu Accueil was to hold onto every gift he received. She wanted him to save every gift so he will not end up like her—old and destitute.[94]

La Vieille was an embittered old woman who blamed men, youth, and old age for her current impoverished condition. She explained:

> Know then, that if only, when I was your age, I had been as wise about the games of Love as I am now! For then I was a very great beauty, but now I must complain and moan when I look at my face, which has lost its charms; and I see the inevitable wrinkles whenever I remember how my beauty made the young men skip. I made them so struggle that it was nothing if not a marvel.

> I was very famous then; my word of my highly renowned beauty
> ran everywhere. At my house there was a crowd so big that no
> man ever saw the like. As I say, if I had been as wise then as I am
> now, I would posses the value of a thousand pounds of sterling
> silver more than I do now, but I acted foolishly. Now, through
> my own wretched act, I am a poor woman. They gave to me,
> and I gave away; I have kept back nothing. Giving has reduced
> me to indigence. I did not remember old age, that has put me in
> such distress. I never thought of poverty. I let time go by just as
> it came, taking no care to spend moderately.[95]

In her youth, La Vieille was a celebrated beauty who had her pick of
any man. Men would line up at her door and lavish her with gifts, money,
and attention. However, she was ignorant and irrational when it came to
love and money. As a young woman, la Vieille never thought about her
financial future. Instead of saving her money and gifts, she squandered
them on an abusive man who did not reciprocate her love. He only used
her for financial gain and left her when everything was spent. Now, she is
a poor, wrinkled old woman whose looks repel men:

> No one is coming today, no one came yesterday, I thought,
> unhappy wretch! I must live in sorrow. My woeful heart should
> have left me. Then, when I saw my door, and even myself, at
> such repose, I wanted to leave the country, for I couldn't endure
> the shame. How could I stand it when handsome young men
> came along, those who formerly had held me so dear that they
> could not tire themselves, and I saw them look at me sideways
> as they passed by, they who had once been my dear guests? They
> went by near me, bounding along without counting me worth
> an egg, even those who had loved me most; they called me a
> wrinkled old woman and worse before they had passed on by.[96]

La Vieille went from being a renowned beauty in her youth to a
shameful, unsightly figure in old age. The countless men who used to line
up at her door with gifts and money now ridicule her because of her old
age. Her former lovers viewed her as a worthless, ugly old woman who
deserved humiliation and disrespect.

Although la Vieille was old, poor, and unattractive, she was wise in
love: "I have so much knowledge upon which I can lecture from a chair

that I could never finish."[97] Her wisdom in love and deceit improved with age and experience. With this knowledge, la Vieille informed the younger generations about using their minds and bodies for the purpose of economic survival and financial security in old age.[98]

The depiction of sexually manipulative old women in medieval literature was not a new concept. In the early first century, the Roman poet, Ovid wrote about a sexually deceptive old woman in his famous work, *Amores*. In the *Amores*, an old woman named Dipsa gives advice to a young, beautiful girl about exploiting men for money and gifts. Hence, the old woman instructed the girl to seduce generous, rich men with her beauty and sweet words. Once she has them in her clutches, the girl should squeeze as many gifts out of them as possible. To keep an admirer interested in her, the old woman advised her to cry, throw a tantrum, or make him jealous. Dipsa told her to follow her advice because "these tactics are guaranteed by a lifetime's experience."[99]

Old Women as Go-Betweens

The portrayal of old women as go-betweens was a familiar theme in medieval literature. However, the depiction of old women as go-betweens was not a new concept in medieval literature. The immensely popular anonymous Latin comedy, *Pamphilus* illustrated a manipulative old woman who tricked a young woman into her home so that she could be seduced by her admirer. *Pamphilus* was written in France between 1100 and 1150. It enjoyed wide readership since it was translated into Old French around 1225, into Venetian dialect around 1250, and into Old Norse some time in the thirteenth century. Around 170 manuscripts of *Pamphilus* exist.[100]

Pamphilus told a tale of a young man (Pamphilus) who was in love with his wealthy, beautiful young neighbor named Galathea. However, Galathea was uninterested in Pamphilus because she did not trust him. She knew of too many men who had deceived women with 'false promises' and 'tricks'.[101] Moreover, she refused to converse with him in public or be alone with him since it would cause scandal and gossip. Since Pamphilus wanted to get together with Galathea, he employed a poor old woman, known as the bawd, to act as a go-between.[102] Pamphilus hired the bawd to serve as a go-between because she was knowledgeable in love: "Nearby lives an old woman, subtle, crafty, a useful handmaiden of the arts of Venus."[103] As a go-between, the bawd tried to persuade Galathea that Pamphilus was the right man for her by exaggerating and lying about his supposed qualities. The old woman described Pamphilus as the most handsome, sweet, generous, wise, honorable, and wealthy man in the city, though in reality, he had neither "shining honor nor great wealth."[104] Furthermore, the bawd told Galathea not to worry about causing shame or gossip, but to be brave in love and enjoy life while she is still young. With the old woman's words of praise and encouragement, Galathea became more interested in Pamphilus.[105]

In order to get Pamphilus and Galathea alone together, the bawd had Pamphilus wait outside her house until she had lured Galathea into her home with apples and nuts. Once Galathea was inside the bawd's house, Pamphilus knocked on the door and entered the house. As Pamphilus was telling Galathea his feelings for her, the bawd excused herself when she heard her neighbor calling out for her. While the old woman was outside, Pamphilus raped Galathea.[106]

According to Galathea, she could not come to love Pamphilus: "You've conquered me, however strongly I resisted, but all hope of love is shattered between us—forever!" Having lost her virginity, Galathea feared that her parents would kick her out of the house since she was now impure.[107]

Galathea blamed the old woman for deceiving her: "She did wrong, that old woman, entrusting me to you. I'll never come here again; she will not deceive me a second time."[108] Galathea further accused the old woman of feigning ignorance:

> It suits you, doesn't it, to pretend that you have no idea what happened [the rape], when everything was done in accord with your plans. As a tree is known by its fruit, so you will be known by your deeds. Apples and nuts—you were deceitful to offer me them when that Pamphilus of yours was right at your door. And your neighbor, she called you so that he would have the opportunity for this, for me to lose my virginity. What else caused you to delay so long out of doors? How well your art concealed your snares. Your art and deceit have run their course; the fleeting hare has fallen into you trap.[109]

The bawd replied:

> I am unjustly accused. Away with all blame for me! I shall clear myself to your satisfaction. This accusation does not accord well with my years, nor do I employ my skill in such evil ways. If

some quarrel arose in your play, how could I be at fault? I was
not even here! Be that as it may, this strife has nothing to do with
me. It wasn't I but your love which inspired it.[110]

Although the bawd had arranged a surprise meeting between the two
(a surprise on Galathea's part), she refused to take the blame. Instead, she
argued that she was just doing her job as a go-between:

Make peace now; it's best for you both. Let this woman be your
wife. Let this man be your husband. Through my aid, you both
now have what you wanted; through me you are happy. Never
forget me![111]

In the romance, *Il Filocolo* (*The Love Afflicted*, c.1336-38), Giovanni
Boccaccio represented a poor, old woman as a go-between. *Il Filocolo*
never shared the same success as Boccaccio's later work, *The Decameron*
(1349-51). There are not many translations or editions of this work. Most
of its editions exist from the sixteenth century (seven editions).[112]

Resembling *Pamphilus*, *Il Filocolo* told a story of a young man in love
with a young noble lady. Boccaccio depicted her as "a young lady in our
city who was very lovely and gracious, noble and rich in wealth and great
in family."[113] Since the young man was too scared to inform the lady of his
feelings, he hired an old woman to act as a go-between. The old woman
was described as "a poor old woman, as shrunken and withered and sorry
in appearance as could be found anywhere."[114]

The young man hired this old woman to act as a go-between because
he had seen her enter the lady's house to beg for alms and return with the
young woman. As a go-between, the old woman informed the lady about
the young man's love for her and vice versa. Thus, the old woman arranged
a clandestine meeting between the young man and lady. However, the
lady's brothers found them together. For attempting to disgrace them, the
brothers offered the young man the following option:

Either we kill you, or you must sleep with both this old woman
and our sister, for a year apiece, and loyally swear that if you
choose to sleep with them for two years and spend the first
with the maiden, that however many times you kiss her or do
anything else with her, you will kiss or do that the same number
of times the second year with the old woman; or if you take

the old woman the first year, however many times you kiss or touch her you will do similarly the second year with the maiden, neither more nor less.[115]

Since the young man did not want to die, he chose to sleep with the two women for the two years. The story does not mention who the young man chose to sleep with first—the young lady or the old woman.[116]

Old Women with Extraordinary Powers

Old women were sometimes portrayed in literature as possessing extraordinary powers. They had the ability to control life and death and transform themselves and others into beautiful, young women or fearless knights. Although they were depicted as unsightly old hags, they were magical women with immense power.

The anonymous English poem, "Sir Gawain and the Green Knight,"(c.1370) featured an ugly, old woman by the name of Morgan le Fay. In the poem, a young knight named Gawain meets a young woman, Lady Bercilak, and an old noble woman, Morgan le Fay, at the lord's castle. He greeted the young lady with a kiss and the aged woman with a low bow. Gawain described Lady Bercilak as, "The fairest of them all in skin, in flesh and complexion, in form and colouring and manners" while Morgan le Fay appeared to him withered with saggy, wrinkled cheeks. The young lady wore a dress that displayed her neck, and had many pearls on her kerchief, while the noble woman:

> Was swathed in a gorget that hid her neck, her swarthy chin was wrapped in chalk-white veils, her forehead enveloped in silk, and she was muffled up everywhere, trellised around with trefoils and rings. Nothing was bare of that lady but her black brows, the eyes and the nose, the naked lips, and those were sour and marvellously bleared. An honourable lady on earth we may call her, by God! Her body was short and thick, her buttocks round and broad; more sweet to taste was that lady with her."[117]

In "Sir Gawain and the Green Knight," the physical body was described as different for the young and the old. Lady Bercilak displayed her neck, while Morgan le Fay was fully covered, except for a portion of her face. Even though Morgan le Fay was recognized as an honorable lady and was shown respect, her physical faults were criticized. According to Gawain, the older woman's face and body were a sore sight for the eyes. Her body was "short and thick," she had a "swarthy" complexion, and her buttocks were "round and broad."[118]

Furthermore, Gawain elaborated more on Morgan le Fay's appearance than Lady Bercilak's appearance. He provided details about the older woman's face, body type and shape, clothing, and the color of her eyebrows and veils, but only fleetingly noted the lady's bare skin, body type, and complexion.[119] The lady's appearance must have been too perfect for words to describe. To Gawain, Lady Bercilak epitomized the ideal woman: young and slender with a fresh complexion and good manners. Conversely, Morgan le Fay represented the undesirable woman: old and fat with wrinkles and saggy skin.

Nonetheless, Morgan le Fay was not only a noble woman, but a powerful sorceress who learned much of her magic from the renowned wizard Merlin. With her magic, Morgan transformed Lord Bercilak into the immortal and undefeatable Green Knight to challenge Gawain's pride. According to Lord Bercilak, Morgan le Fay had the ability to cut anyone down to size: "No one possesses such high pride; whom she cannot make very tame."[120] She sent the Green Knight to test the Round Table's valor, to outwit Gawain, and to frighten Queen Guinevere by having him (the Green Knight) talk to her while holding his own severed head in his hands. Morgan le Fay was a commanding figure who had the ability to control life and death and outdo anyone, including Gawain, with her magical powers.[121]

Geoffrey Chaucer's "The Wife of Bath's Tale" from *The Canterbury Tales* (c.1385-1400) and John Gower's "The Tale of Florent" from his famous work, *Confessio Amantis* (*The Lover's Confession*, c.1386-90) closely resembled each other in content. Both works told a tale of a young knight whose life was in the hands of an old woman with extraordinary powers. This similarity was due in part to the friendship between Geoffrey Chaucer and John Gower. As friends and contemporaries, Chaucer and Gower often influenced each other's writings. In fact, John Gower dedicated *Confessio Amantis* to Geoffrey Chaucer and to Richard II of England (who commissioned the book), while Chaucer dedicated his *Troilus and Criseyde* (c.1385) to Gower and to philosopher Ralph Strode. Over forty manuscripts of Gower's *Confessio Amantis* are known to exist. The earliest known manuscript dates from 1390.[122]

In "The Wife of Bath's Tale," a knight in King Arthur's Court was charged with raping a young girl, while in "The Tale of Florent," the knight was charged with killing another knight. In both stories, the knight was sentenced to die. However, the knight could escape death if he could answer one question. If the knight answered the question correctly then his life would be spared, but if he answered it incorrectly then he would die. The question was posed by (in Chaucer's version) King Arthur's wife, Guinevere and by (in Gower's version) the grandmother of the slain knight. They wanted to know what women most desired. Therefore, the knight was given a year and a day to find the answer.[123]

In both stories, women determined the knight's punishment and fate. It was they who possessed the answer to what women most desired. With this knowledge, they exerted power over men.

While on his quest, the knight encountered an old woman in the forest. In "The Wife of Bath's Tale," the old woman was described as "the ugliest person you could imagine."[124] In "The Tale of Florent," the old woman was depicted in much greater detail:

> He saw the old hag where she sat, and a more loathsome thing was that than ever met the human eye. Her nose was flat, her eyebrows high; tiny her eyes, and deeply set; with dripping tears her cheeks were wet, and wrinkled as an empty skin, and they hung down upon her chin; her lips had shrunk, she was so old. She had no beauties to behold: her forehead narrow, her locks hoar, her shoulders curving, her neck short, such as no pleasure could support; her body thick by no means small; and shortly to describe her all, never a limb without a lack.[125]

The old woman was portrayed in a highly unflattering manner. Both authors concentrated on her physical faults. Chaucer described the old woman as hideous, while Gower depicted her as a fat, disgusting old hag who had loose, wrinkly skin, matted hair, small eyes, and withered lips.

Although the old woman was physically repulsive, she possessed great wisdom: "we old folk know a great many things."[126] Thus, the young knight asked the old woman for some advice. She agreed to answer his question under one condition—if he promised to do whatever she asked of him. He did not want to die so he promised to do whatever she wanted in exchange for the answer. Hence, the old woman replied to his question:

"women wish to have sovereignty over their husbands as well as their lovers and to be in authority over them."[127] The old woman's wisdom made her a powerful figure. She held the answer to the question that the knight needed to survive. Her control over the knight's life placed him in a vulnerable position. In turn, she used his helplessness to her advantage.

After answering the question correctly, Guinevere/the slain knight's grandmother set him free. In return for saving his life, the old woman asked him to marry her. At first, the knight tried to get out of marrying her. He offered her all of his possessions, but she refused. Ultimately, the knight agreed to marry her since he had made a promise. Even though the knight was repelled by the old woman's age, looks, and poverty, he did see some advantages to the marriage: he could send her to an island where no one knew her or she could die soon of old age.[128]

The young knight married the old woman in secret without any festivities. For the rest of the day, he hid from her and at night, he avoided her in bed. Therefore, the old woman asked him why he was acting so strangely towards her on their wedding night. He explained to her that he was repulsed by her old age, ugliness, and low status. The old woman replied that she may be old and hideous, but she will always be faithful to him: "dirt and age are the best guardians of chastity."[129]

Although the old woman was wise, kind, and loyal, the knight could not see beyond her age and grotesque physical appearance. Since the knight was miserable with her, the old woman gave him a choice:

> Either to have me old and ugly for the rest of my life, but a faithful, obedient wife; or else to have me young and fair, and take your chance with all the men who will resort because of me to your house—or to some other place perhaps![130]

The knight replied:

> My lady and my love, and my dearest wife, I trust myself to your wise guidance; do you yourself choose whichever may be the most pleasing and honorable for both of us. I care not which of the two you choose, for whatever pleases you will satisfy me.[131]

With these words, the old woman transformed into a beautiful, young woman because the knight allowed her to make the decision. Therefore, the knight, along with his young and faithful wife, lived happily ever after.[132]

Poor Old Women

Old women were frequently portrayed in such medieval literary works as *Pamphilus*, *Le Roman de la Rose*, *Il Filocolo*, "The Wife of Bath's Tale," and "The Tale of Florent" as poor and pitiful. Their poverty was usually emphasized by their pathetic appearance, such as, the old woman from "The Wife of Bath's Tale" and "The Tale of Florent" and by their stories of financial hardship, like la Vieille's from *Le Roman de la Rose*.

Besides "The Wife of Bath's Tale," Geoffrey Chaucer depicted two more impoverished women in "The Nun's Priest's Tale" and "The Friar's Tale" in his *Canterbury Tales*. In "The Nun's Priest's Tale," Chaucer briefly described the old widow as "a poor widow somewhat advanced in age" with little property or money.[133] She lived in a tiny cottage with her two daughters and some farm animals. She ate sparse meals and had no need for extravagant things she could not afford. Overall, the widow lived a humble existence.[134]

"The Friar's Tale" concerns a couple of thieves (one was a summoner who greatly misused his power and the other was the devil himself) who tried to trick an old widow out of her money. The summoner described the old woman as a miserly "old bag who'd almost as soon cut her throat as give up a penny of her goods." He also called her an 'old cow' and an 'old harridan' in order to stress her age and his disgust towards her.[135]

To swindle the old widow out of her money, the summoner pretended to have a writ of summons for her to attend court. Since she was too old and sick to go to court, the summoner stated that he would acquit her for twelve pence instead. Clearly shocked, the old woman declared:

> 'Twelve pence!' she cried. 'Were you to give me the whole wide world, I haven't got twelve pence in my pocket. Can't you see I'm old and poor? Show charity to a poor wretch like me!'[136]

Showing no mercy, the summoner took her frying pan as payment. The old woman was so upset about the situation that she wished the devil would take the summoner and the frying pan to hell, which he gladly did.[137]

The summoner in "The Friar's Tale" tried to take advantage of the widow because she was old, poor, and vulnerable. Since the old widow lived alone and unprotected, the summoner thought he could barge into her home on false charges and demand money. He made up the summons story because he knew she was too old and sick to attend court and would probably pay the fine instead. Even though the old woman did not have any money, the summoner was adamant on taking everything she owned: "I've no mind to repent for anything I've had of you—I'd sooner take your smock and every stitch from your back!"[138] Hence, he was keen on making the old woman's life even more wretched and impoverished.

Useless Old Women

In addition to Chaucer's representation of poor, vulnerable old women, women past their reproductive years were sometimes depicted as useless, insignificant, and/or limited in their helpfulness. In the renowned epic poem, *Willehalm* (c.1212-17), the German poet, Wolfram von Eschenbach wrote about a determined old woman who was discouraged by her son from participating in battle because she was old. There are over seventy manuscripts of *Willehalm* in existence. The manuscripts date from the thirteenth, fourteenth, and fifteenth centuries.[139]

When the title character Willehalm planned a religious war against the Saracens, his old mother, Countess Irmschart of Pavia, offered him aid, but expressed some doubt to her helpfulness when she stated: "What am I good for after all, old woman that I am?"[140] Though Irmschart considered old age as an impediment, she still wanted to help her son. She wished to provide him with money and an army and was willing to wield the sword herself:

> I shall wear armour myself. I am a woman strong enough to bear
> arms at your side. The brave man, not the coward, will be able to
> see me with you. I shall strike blows with my swords.[141]

Despite his mother's determination to fight, Willehalm did not believe that she should participate in battle. Willehalm explained:

> Send my father to fight, for he can take command of an army,
> and he will fight where it is necessary. A helmet is not meant for
> you [Irmschart] nor other weapons, nor a shield. But if it is not
> asking too much, Madam, give your support as you offered it
> [material support].[142]

Willehalm wanted his old father to fight, but not his old mother. He did not specify the reason why, but it was probably because she was an old woman since he did not have a problem with his old father fighting or having his wife Giburc and her ladies wield a sword. For instance, when the Saracens were outside Willehalm and Giburc's fortress, she and her ladies put on armor and armed themselves with swords and crossbows:

> Now Lady Giburc stood with upraised sword ready to defend herself, as if looking for combat, and with her stood Stephen, her chaplain, and her maidens attired in armour. Neither the maiden Karpite fighting before Laurent, nor Kamille of Volcan was armed so well. But Giburc had not fought on horseback. This tale attributes other brave deeds to her, saying that she shot the crossbow, hurled huge stones, and that her defence was marked by clever tactics. She propped up her dead soldiers on the battlements dressed in their armour and manipulated them so skillfully that it inspired fear in the enemy outside, who were erecting siege equipment against her.[143]

Willehalm did not mind having his wife and her ladies defending the fortress. In fact, he wanted them to continue their support:

> He [Willehalm] addressed the others who were still alive with Giburc in the fortress, saying that they would always participate with him in whatever he might possess, be they woman or man, young ladies or other maidens.[144]

Even though Willehalm's old father and his wife wielded the sword, his old mother was excluded from participating in the fight against the Saracens. Instead, she was only needed for material support. Her hopes of fighting in her son's war were soon quickly dashed.

In the famous satirical work, *The Decameron* (*Ten Days*), Giovanni Boccaccio portrayed old women as valueless and unimportant. Boccaccio wrote *The Decameron* between 1349-51 during the Black Death. The oldest surviving manuscript dates from 1368. More than ten editions of *The Decameron* were printed in the fifteenth century and seventy-seven were printed in the sixteenth century.[145]

In the tenth story of the fifth day of *The Decameron*, Boccaccio wrote about a frustrated young wife whose husband did not take any interest in her. Since she was young, beautiful, and rich, the wife did not understand why her husband ignored her. To solve this problem, she sought the advice of an old woman. The old woman told her to have numerous love affairs and enjoy life while she was still young. She added that old age only brings grief. The old woman complained:

> And what a devil are we women good for, once we are old, save to keep the ashes about the fire pot? . . . God knoweth what chagrin I feel. With men it is not so; they are born apt for a thousand things, not for this alone, and most part of them are of much more account old than young; but women are born into the world for nothing but to do this [have sex] and bear children, and it is for this that they are prized . . . when we grow old, nor husband nor other will look at us; nay, they send us off to the kitchen to tell tales to the cat and count the pots and pans; and what is worse, they tag rhymes on us and say, "Tidbits for wenches young; Gags for the old wife's tongue."[146]

According to the old woman, a woman's value was limited to two functions—sex and reproduction.[147] Her most prized asset, having children, was restricted to her reproductive years. The old woman asserted that women were recognized only during their reproductive years. They were disregarded in their post-menopausal years. Women past their childbearing years were not useful for anything, except being ignored or ridiculed by their husbands. To Boccaccio, once a woman reached menopause, her worth significantly decreased.[148]

Boccaccio, however, believed that a man's value was not limited to a particular period or function. Men, young and old, were esteemed for doing countless things throughout their lives. To him, a man's ability to do "a thousand things" only improved with age, hence, making him more revered in his old age.[149]

Medieval literary writers held mainly negative attitudes toward old women. Old women were viewed by Geoffrey Chaucer, John Gower, and the anonymous author of *Les Quinze Joies de Mariage* as impoverished old hags or as sexually manipulative bawds. Other popular medieval writers, such as Wolfram von Eschenbach and Giovanni Boccaccio perceived post-menopausal women as useless and/or limited in their helpfulness. To them, a woman's worth was confined to their reproductive years. Jean de Meun characterized old women as repulsive creatures whose looks repel men. As go-betweens, they were portrayed as sexually experienced women who were knowledgeable in the art of sexual deception. Their wisdom in love and betrayal made them threatening, dangerous, and powerful figures in medieval literature. Nonetheless, literary attitudes toward post-menopausal women have often diverged from evidence of lived lives. There have been a number of instances of post-menopausal women who have contradicted literary stereotypes by taking up positions of authority and independence.

CHAPTER 4

THE LIVES OF POST-MENOPAUSAL WOMEN IN THE HIGH AND LATE MIDDLE AGES

Old women were typically depicted in a disapproving manner in various didactic and literary works in the High and Late Middle Ages. They were characterized in these works as undesirable, unable to love, impoverished, useless, foolish, deviant, dangerous, childlike, and weak in mind, body, and spirit. Nonetheless, the chapter investigates the lives of several post-menopausal women (abbesses, noble women, peasant women, and widows) who disregarded these stereotypes and assumed positions of power and independence. These women continued to lead active lives for as long as possible.

Abbess

The German abbess, Hildegard of Bingen (1098-1179) was an accomplished woman of her age. She lived during a period when women experienced greater freedom and independence in the Church than they would in the following century. In 1150, at the age of fifty-two, Hildegard founded a convent on Mount St. Rupert at Bingen (Germany). Before the move, she was abbess (1136-50) of Disibodenberg, a shared community of monks and nuns. At Disibodenberg, the nun's quarters were crowded and the abbot controlled their wealth from donations and dowries. Hildegard decided to set up a new house because she sought better living conditions and financial independence. She bought land near Rupertsberg and established a new convent for her nuns. There, the nuns were no longer under the authority of the monks and held their properties independently.[150]

Beginning in 1158, at the age of sixty, Hildegard conducted the first of four preaching tours around Germany. Her first, second, and third preaching tours occurred in Bamberg (1158), Trier and Lorraine (1160) and Siegburg and Cologne (1161-63). In 1170-71, at the age of seventy-three, Hildegard completed her fourth and final tour through Swabia. She traveled by boat in her first three tours and by land during her fourth. Although she suffered from poor health, she possessed enough energy and zeal to make these excursions around Germany.[151]

As the convent at Rupertsberg grew, there was need for more room. In 1165, when she was sixty-seven, Hildegard founded another a at Eibingen. She served as abbess at Rupertsberg and Eibingen until her death at the age of eighty-one.[152]

Noble Women

Another commanding figure in the twelfth century was Matilda (1102-67), daughter of Henry I of England, empress of Germany, countess of Anjou, and the mother of Henry II of England. When Henry II became king in 1154, he delegated some of his power to his mother Matilda. This delegation of authority can be observed by an 1155 mandate issued by Henry addressed to his bailiffs, justices, and counts of Normandy concerning the land of the church of Fécamp. Henry ended the mandate with the following statement: "Unless you do it, let my lady and mother the empress see that it is done."[153]

Furthermore, Matilda acted as deputy in his duchy of Normandy while he was away. In 1154, while Henry was away in Aquitaine, Matilda, along with the archbishop of Rouen, confirmed the appointment of Robert of Torigny as the elected abbot of Mont-Saint-Michel. Robert of Torigny was an abbot and historian who noted this event in his work *Chronicle*.[154]

Independently, and with her son, Matilda founded and patronized abbeys, issued Norman and English charters and writs, and heard legal cases in Normandy. In 1159, she issued an executive writ to the sheriff of Herefordshire (England), commanding him, under the authority of herself and her son, to ensure that there were no legal proceedings enacted against the monks of Reading in regard to their lands. Matilda and Henry II wanted to protect the monks' lands because Reading was a royal abbey where her father, Henry I, was buried. She continued to advise and perform administrative duties for her son until her death in 1167 at the age of sixty-five.[155]

Empress Matilda's daughter-in-law, Eleanor of Aquitaine (1122-1204) was another remarkable and influential woman who gained power as she aged. Eleanor was the first wife of Louis VII of France, and then the wife of Henry II of England, the mother of Richard I and John I of England, the duchess of Aquitaine and Normandy, and the countess of Anjou. In 1173, at the age of fifty-one, Eleanor and her sons, Henry, Richard, and Geoffrey, rebelled against Henry II because he would not grant his sons autonomous control of their allotted lands nor give his son, Henry, who was crowned king during his father's lifetime, any kind of sovereign power.[156]

During Eleanor's feud with Henry in 1173, the French poet and theologian, Peter of Blois, at the request of his patron, Rotrou of Warwick, the Archbishop of Rouen, wrote a letter to Eleanor demanding her to return to her husband or else face dire consequences. Throughout his letter, Peter of Blois denounced Eleanor for leaving her husband and influencing her children to rebel against him. He wrote:

> Pious Queen, most illustrious Queen, we all of us deplore, and are united in our sorrow, that you, a prudent wife if ever there was one, should have parted from your husband . . . Still more terrible is the fact that you should have made the fruits of your union with our Lord King rise up against their father . . . Before events carry us to a dire conclusion, return with your sons to the husband whom you must obey and with whom it is your duty to live . . . Either you will return to your husband, or else, by canon law, we shall be compelled and forced to bring the censure of the Church to bear on you.[157]

After winning the rebellion, Henry II had Eleanor imprisoned in 1174 for disloyalty and for conspiring against him. She remained a prisoner in various castles until her husband's death fifteen years later in 1189.[158] Once freed from confinement, Eleanor became even more powerful and influential in the political realm.

Eleanor exerted immense power and dedication in advancing her sons' interests, particularly Richard's, her favorite son. In 1189, she oversaw Richard's coronation and helped him organize the Crusade. A year later, Eleanor traveled to Spain to arrange Richard's marriage to Berengaria of Navarre. Eleanor and Berengaria then traveled to Sicily to meet with

Richard.[159] During this time, the contemporary chronicler of Richard I, Richard of Devizes described Eleanor as:

> A matchless woman, beautiful and chaste, powerful and modest, meek and eloquent, which is rarely to be met with in a woman; who was sufficiently advanced in years to have two husbands and two sons crowned kings, still indefatigable for every understanding, whose power was the admiration of her age.[160]

Richard of Devizes further noted: "even now unwearied by any task, and provoked wonder by her stamina."[161]

Clearly, Eleanor's age did not affect her mental and physical prowess. She virtually ruled England while Richard was away on a Crusade and held for ransom in Germany. The thirteenth century chronicler, Matthew Paris described Eleanor as an "exceedingly respected and beloved" monarch who ruled England "with great wisdom and popularity."[162] Throughout 1193, Eleanor governed England and raised money for Richard's ransom. After raising enough funds, Eleanor traveled to Germany to pay off Richard's captors.[163]

In 1194, then seventy-two, Eleanor retired to the abbey of Fontevraud. Following Richard's death in 1199, Eleanor left the abbey to secure the English throne for John. During this time, she traveled around France receiving homage, settling disputes, granting charters, hearing appeals, and dispensing lands and castles.[164]

After becoming king, John continued to receive advice from Eleanor about preserving peace between England and France. In hopes of bringing peace between John I and Philip II, Eleanor crossed the Pyrenees into Spain in 1200 to arrange the marriage between her granddaughter (and John's niece), Blanche of Castile, and Louis, the son of Philip II. After the marriage arrangements were completed, Eleanor returned to the abbey of Fontevraud where she died in 1204 at the age of eighty-two.[165]

Like her grandmother, Blanche of Castile (1188-1252) was a forceful woman who was determined to protect her son's interests and inheritance. When her husband, Louis VIII of France died in 1226, Blanche served as regent for her twelve-year-old son Louis IX until he came of age eight years later. In 1248 at the age of sixty, Blanche once again served as regent when Louis IX joined a crusade. As regent, Blanche was a skilled administrator who was actively involved in the political sphere of the French realm. She continued her role as regent until her death in 1252 at the age of sixty-four.[166]

The thirteenth century chronicler of Louis IX, Guillaume de Nangis paid respect to the memory of Blanche of Castile with the following statement: "She was the wisest of all women of her time, and all good things came to the realm of France while she was alive."[167]

Another woman who led an active life as she aged was Countess Marguerite of Flanders and Hainaut (1202-80). In 1244, Marguerite inherited Flanders when her older sister, Jeanne, died. From 1244-78, Marguerite actively ruled Flanders. She was involved in diplomatic relations between France, Germany, England, and the Low Countries. Moreover, Marguerite stimulated international trade by transforming Bruges into a major international port. She expanded the canal system, suppressed urban uprisings, minted new coins, supported writers and poets, founded Dominican houses, and had new public buildings built in Flanders. In 1278, Marguerite abdicated as countess of Flanders in favor of her son Guy of Dampierre, but continued to rule Hainaut until her death in 1280 at the age of seventy-eight.[168]

In the early fourteenth-century French village of Montaillou, according to inquisitional records, there was a post-menopausal woman who remained sexually active and defied the Church and her family in order to be with her young lover. Béatrice de Planissoles was a twice widowed noble woman who was "past the change of life" when she first met and fell in love with Barthélemy Amilhac, a young parish priest, in 1316. Béatrice accused him of bewitching her:

> I have never committed the sin of sorcery. But I think the priest Barthélemy did cast a spell on me, for I loved him too passionately; and yet when I met him I was already past the menopause.[169]

Their affair caused much scandal and gossip among the villagers because she was an old widow and her lover was a young priest. Béatrice's brothers were so angry with her that she was terrified they would do her bodily harm. Furthermore, the Church was on a campaign to end the clergy's custom of living with women. By forming a papal Inquisition, the church tried to enforce clerical celibacy in regions such as Montaillou.[170]

In order to escape village gossip, furious relatives, and the papal Inquisition, Béatrice and Barthélemy left Montaillou and moved to Palhars, an isolated diocese in the Pyrenees. At Palhars, priests were still allowed to live with women, but for a price. The bishop gave the diocese permission to continue this practice in return for money. There, Béatrice and Barthélemy lived together for a year until they parted ways.[171] Their separation was mainly due to Béatrice's Catharism. He was afraid of being discovered by the Inquisition for his involvement with a heretic. When Barthélemy was seized and interrogated by the Inquisition in 1320, he described Béatrice as a "wicked old woman" and a "heretic".[172]

Straying from convention, Béatrice de Planissoles fell subject to malicious gossip and resentful attitudes. She was scorned by those around her (i.e. her family and her village) because she deviated from what was considered age-appropriate behavior. Béatrice embodied many sexual and moral taboos: she was a sexually active post-menopausal widow who was living with a younger man who happened to be a priest. This type of sexual behavior was repeatedly condemned by medieval writers as inappropriate and immoral.

Peasant Women

In addition to research on the eminent lives of abbesses, queens, and countesses, there is evidence of ordinary peasant women who have remained physically active and carried out their daily routines for as long as they were capable. The fourteenth-century Bedfordshire (England) coroners' rolls have provided some examples of this. For instance, an old and frail widow named Mariot rose from her bed to fetch a pitcher of water from a well, but fell in and died. In addition, the coroners' rolls reported a case of a child drowning while under the care of a blind old woman. In 1334, a woman in her seventies named Isabella, fell from a ladder and died while attempting to get some straw to build a fire. In another case, a woman who was around the age of sixty stood on a tree limb next to a well in order to gather fruit, but fell in after the tree limb broke. In 1356, after a tiring day of gleaning the fields for grain, Agnes Watrot, who was in her fifties, returned home and fell asleep without putting out her candle. A fire broke out and Agnes burned to death.[173]

Widows

In contrast to the literary image of the poor, worthless old woman, some women, particularly widows, exerted considerable influence and independence in their advanced years. Unlike dependent wives and semi-dependent daughters, widows were no longer under their husbands' or fathers' authority. Widowhood brought a host of new opportunities and responsibilities that were typically denied to wives and daughters. As householders and landholders, widows independently engaged in social, legal, and economic activities. As a widow, she could sue or be sued, borrow and lend money, make contracts on her own, arrange marriages for her children, and make her own decision about remarriage and whom to marry.[174] In the case of the French village of Montaillou and the English manor of Brigstock, a woman's standing in the domestic and public spheres improved with age while an old man's position declined.

Contrary to the literary image, old widows were not always impoverished, pitiful, and defenseless. A widow's economic condition depended on how much property she brought into the marriage (through inheritance, purchase, or dowry) and her husband's property. Under English common law, a widow was entitled to one-third to one-half of her husband's property for life. Her dower right was legally recognized and protected. Feudal lords and the courts were compelled to acknowledge a widow's dower right even if her husband left debts or bequeathed her portion of the property to another. In addition, a woman who owned land prior to marriage resumed full ownership of the land when her husband died.[175]

This meant noble and aristocratic widows were financially secure in their old age. Because of the low life expectancy of noble men during the High and Late Middle Ages, noble women commonly inherited great fiefs. Some noble women, such as Eleanor of Aquitaine and Marguerite of Flanders, continued to exert power over their feudal territories until they were quite old.[176]

Besides noble women, peasant widows were usually provided for in their old age, at least in the case of England. Husbands made different kinds of provisions for their wives through wills and manorial court agreements. These provisions included: bequeathing their wives the income from a part or all of the property for life, providing them with some land and housing, or making sure that their sons cared for them. In the wills of numerous English and French peasants, a widow was allowed to live in the family house with her son, but if she did not want to live with him then he had to provide her with another house.[177] Barbara Hanawalt's study of the late medieval peasantry in Bedfordshire, England, focused on wills of 235 males whose wives survived them. Hanawalt discovered that sixty-three percent of these women received the home tenement for life, fifteen percent were given land other than their home tenement, five percent received their dowry, five percent were given a separate home, three percent possessed the tenement until their oldest son reached maturity, three percent were given the house, but not the lands, three percent were allowed a room in the house, and two percent were given a dower of one-third of the property. Additionally, fifty-two percent of these women were left money, animals, household goods, and the remains of the property after the debts were paid.[178]

Unfortunately, not all widows were adequately provided for in their old age. Poor women without property, such as the widows of wage earners, usually continued to work for as long as they could or were reduced to begging. Still, there were many charitable organizations in the Middle Ages that aided the poor. Religious houses, churches, guilds, and the community often provided assistance to those in need.[179]

Although some old widows were poor, vulnerable, and dependent on charity, there were others who exerted significant power and independence in their old age. For instance, Judith M. Bennett's *Women in the Medieval English Countryside: Gender and Household in Brigstock Before the Plague* and Emmanuel Le Roy Ladurie's *Montaillou: The Promised Land of Error* provide a glimpse into the legal, social, and economic lives of old peasant widows in medieval England and France. Both historians found that with age, women gained influence and esteem in their communities as men lost command and respect in their old age.

In *Women in the Medieval English Countryside: Gender and Household in Brigstock Before the Plague* (1287-1348), Judith Bennett examined one hundred and one unmarried widows living on the manor of Brigstock, in Northhamptonshire, England.[180] She observed that nearly all widows in Brigstock remained independent heads of households until they died since few remarried and few made provisions for retirement. Although half of the widows in Brigstock were publicly inactive, the other half remained active in the community. The widows who remained publicly active in Brigstock independently bought, sold, traded, and leased land to others. In addition, they answered for their own crimes, resolved disputes at court, and made contracts on their own.[181]

According to Bennett's study, several widows in Brigstock remained socially, economically, and publicly vigorous in their old age.[182] For instance, Emma Sepheride (widowed for over twenty years since 1302) was a widow who remained economically active in Brigstock. As a widow, Emma went to court unaccompanied, managed her landholdings, sold ale and bread, and remained independent of her children. Even though Emma Sepheride granted some of her lands to her sons in exchange for a cartload of hay each year, she still administered other lands on her own. She also provided a house for her two daughters. The preceding actions imply that she held some financial control over her children's lives.[183]

Similar to Emma Sepheride, Matilda Cocus (widowed for over twelve years since 1302) remained independent of her children. She continued to manage her lands with the help of her servants and made frequent court appearances.[184]

Another widow, Alice Avice, a wife for twenty-four years and a widow for sixteen years (widowed in 1316), continued to manage her landholdings and participate in legal matters. As a wife, Alice had usually gone to court accompanied by her husband. As a widow, she regularly attended court alone in order to pay rent on her land, buy and sell lands, answer numerous charges relating to property ownership, and to initiate or respond to various complaints against other villagers. She also broadened her social contacts during widowhood. Throughout Alice's twenty-four years of marriage, she amassed a court network of twenty-two contacts with fourteen people. In her sixteen years of widowhood, she amassed a court network of thirty-four contacts with twenty-five people.[185]

Men, however, participated less in the public sphere of Brigstock as they grew older. Judith Bennett examined the political lives of five men throughout five decades in Brigstock. For each decade, she counted how many times each man appeared in court as pledgers and officers. According to Bennett, the five men most frequently served as pledgers and officers during their second and third decades of court activity. However, their appearances became less frequent in their fourth and fifth decades of court activity. However, their appearances in court declined during their fourth and fifth decades. Thus, the five men gradually withdrew from court activities as they aged.[186]

Another man who slowly withdrew from political and public life as he aged was Henry Kroyl of Brigstock. Henry Kroyl served as a court officer twenty-three times between 1309-19. However, after his son's marriage in 1319, he ceased his official duties.[187]

Akin to Judith Bennett's case study of Brigstock, Emmanual Le Roy Ladurie's *Montaillou: The Promised Land of Error* (1294-1324) found that women in the southern French village of Montaillou gained respect as they aged while a man's standing diminished with age. In Montaillou, old men were much rarer than old women. The shortage of old men and an excess of old women in Montaillou was partly due to the sizeable age difference between men and women at marriage. Men normally married around the age of twenty-five while women usually married between the ages of fourteen and eighteen.[188]

In Montaillou, men in their 30's and 40's were considered physically robust and in their prime of life, but after the age of 50, they were regarded as old and worthless. In a peasant community where strenuous labor was typical, men were valued for their physical strength. Once a man was old and no longer physically strong, his prestige declined.[189] Furthermore, a man's status further diminished when he retired from heading the household. He usually retired from heading the household when his son and heir married. When he retired, his authority would transmit to his son.[190] For instance, the households of Pons Clergue and Bernard Rives were headed and governed by their grown sons. When Bernard Rives' daughter Guillemette asked to borrow a mule, he replied: "I dare do nothing without my son's approval. Come back tomorrow, and he will lend you the mule."[191] Clearly, Bernard did not carry much power in his son's household.

In contrast to the old men of Montaillou, a woman's standing in her family and community improved with age, especially after the age of fifty. Why was that? Le Roy Ladurie believed that menopause brought power and respect to women since "she ceased to be regarded as a sex object."[192] Historian, Shulamith Shahar further elaborated on Le Roy Ladurie's theory:

> Once a woman was no longer a sexual object, she could deal more
> freely with the men of her stratum and with her subordinates,
> and that the latter were less offended by having to obey her
> commands than if she were a young woman.[193]

Once they were no longer seen as a sexual or a procreative object, menopausal and post-menopausal women were freer to participate in society.[194]

Therefore, in Montaillou, elderly women were esteemed for their numerous roles as mothers, mothers-in-law, and grandmothers: they arranged marriages for their children, aided their daughters and daughters-in-law in managing the household, took care of the grandchildren, and provided advice. When a woman's husband (or the male head of household) died, she would sometimes become head of the household and assume the powerful and revered role of matriarch. The matriarchs of Montaillou were bestowed with the honorable title of 'Na', which meant madame or mistress. One matriarch, known as 'Her Grace, Madame Guillemette', went back to her maiden name Maury after her husband Bernard Marty died. Her two grown sons, Jean and Arnaud were also known by their mother's surname. After her husband's death, Guillemette and her two sons moved into a new house where she headed the household. It can be suggested that she played a dominant role over her sons' lives. She remained head of household and accepted or rejected proposed marriages for each of her adult sons.[195]

There were several matriarchs in Montaillou who held commanding positions in their advanced years. For example, Na Roqua, Guillemette "Belote", and Mengarde Clergue were old matriarchs and friends who came from the leading families of Monatillou. They were aggressive in gaining converts for the Cathar religion and sent food to heretics who were imprisoned by the Inquisition (see chapter 1). Mengarde Clergue was successful in converting her widowed friend Raymonde Guilhou to Catharism. Na Roqua was one of the mothers of the Cathar church and served as a consultant to the heads of families. Another old matriarch, Na Ferriola owned a house and employed shepherds to look after her flock of goats. Na Ferreria was a well-known eye healer from the neighboring village of Prades d'Aillon. People from Montaillou would travel to Prades d'Aillon in order to see her. The women of Montaillou remained energetic and influential in their old age.[196]

The women discussed in the preceding pages did not fit the common literary stereotype of being worthless and physically and mentally weak. In fact, many post-menopausal women, such as Hildegard of Bingen, Eleanor of Aquitaine, and the women of Brigstock and Montaillou wielded substantial power and independence in their old age. Old women, particularly widows, frequently acted as heads of households, owned property, and participated in social, legal, and economic activities. Their status as independent householders and landholders brought them more on par with men in the political and economic realm. As demonstrated in the case studies of Brigstock and Montaillou, men were more likely than women to withdraw from public life and depreciate in value after the age of fifty. Age brought power and reverence to women. They were venerated members of their families and communities for their immeasurable abilities and functions.

CONCLUSION

The period of 1100-1400 experienced a decline in power and status for women. It witnessed the rise of Church power, the Albigensian Crusade and Inquisition, the Black Death, and economic changes that altered women's work roles in the post-plague years. These events affected the lives of women in work, religion, and society. In medieval didactic and prescriptive works and literature, writers perceived the aging process, old age, and post-menopausal women in a disparaging manner. They criticized old women for their deviant ways and venomous bodies. Authors often characterized post-menopausal women as lusty, spurned by love/lover, as go-betweens, having extraordinary powers, poor, and useless. Nevertheless, there have been several examples of post-menopausal women during this period who defied literary stereotypes and conventions and took on positions of power and independence.

From my sources, I have found that discourses on post-menopausal women in the High and Late Middle Ages were dissimilar to how they actually lived their lives. The sources differed in terms of attitudes and perceptions regarding post-menopausal women in the Middle Ages. Didactic and prescriptive works and literature tended to display attitudes that were more negative, satiric, and pessimistic than sources on lived lives.

This difference may be due to the fact that men wrote every didactic/ prescriptive and literary work examined in this book, except for Hildegard of Bingen's *Scivias*. Negative attitudes concerning post-menopausal women did not originate nor conclude in the Middle Ages. In fact, many medieval writings were heavily inspired by Greek and Roman attitudes in relation to post-menopausal women, such as the writings of Aristotle and Ovid. Attitudes concerning women were influenced, in part, by the ancient Greek notion that women were inferior in body and mind. Thus, medieval writers carried on with the long tradition of depicting post-menopausal women in a pessimistic and misogynistic manner.

Furthermore, a large number of medieval women, especially peasant women, were illiterate and therefore, unable to read writings on post-menopausal women. Since books were rare and expensive before the invention of the printing press, literate women may not have had access to these writings.

Moreover, many medieval didactic and prescriptive works were moralistic and dictatorial in tone. They sought to instruct the reader on the accepted norms of society, such as the accepted age when women lost their ability to love and condemned women who did not conform to age-appropriate behavior. These writings tended to define old women based on convention. Thus, one cannot always take them literally as descriptions of behavior.

As works of fiction, literature can reflect or distort reality. Several medieval works of literature, such as Giovanni Boccaccio's *The Decameron* and Geoffrey Chaucer's *The Canterbury Tales* were humorous and satirical. They sought to amuse the reader. In turn, their writings tended to stereotype, exaggerate, and ridicule post-menopausal women in relation to their mind and body, sexuality, and status. Therefore, these works should be taken more figuratively than literally.

In contrast to didactic and prescriptive works and literature, sources on lived lives viewed post-menopausal women in a more positive manner. Most of the sources on lived lives consisted of legal records, such as tax, court, manorial, and coroners' rolls. These sources often recorded women's activities in society. Legal sources cited women as householders, landholders, and participants in social, economic, and legal transactions.

The attitudes expressed by medieval didactic/prescriptive and literary writers concerning post-menopausal women were more unsympathetic and demeaning than respectful and optimistic. They constantly emphasized their faults and criticized their abilities. To them, a woman past menopause should withdraw from life and become virtually non-existent since her main purpose in life (having children) was finished. They were viewed as useless old hags who corrupted the younger generations, deceived men, and mistreated their husbands.

Despite negative discourse and a decline in power and status for women in Europe during the period of 1100-1400, there is evidence of post-menopausal women participating in numerous activities. The women discussed in the preceding pages did not retire meekly into the shadows once they reached menopause, but continued to be physically vigorous, mentally alert, and sexually active. Age did not prevent these women from governing countries, managing households, owning property, making business transactions, performing everyday tasks, forming relationships, and participating in their communities. Hence, a medieval woman's significance did not cease at menopause, but progressed with age, resulting in new roles and opportunities.

APPENDIX

STAGES OF LIFE

Bernard de Gordon's medical work, *De Conservatione Vitae Humanae* (c.1307-08):
1. *Aetas pueritiae*—from birth to age 14
2. *Aetas inventuties*—14 to 35
3. ***Aetas senestutis* (old age)—35 to the end of life**[197]

Bartholomaeus Anglicus' scientific encyclopedia, *De Rerum Proprietatibus* (c.1230-40):
1. Adolescentia—0 to 26 or 30
2. Juventus—26 or 30 to 45 or 50
3. **Senectus (old age)—45 or 50 to 60**
4. **Senium (extreme old age)—60 to 70**[198]

Aldebrandin of Siena's medical treatise, *Le Régime du Corps* (c.1256-57):
1. *Adolescentia*—from birth to 25 or 30
2. *Juventus*—25 or 30 to 40 or 45
3. ***Senectus* (old age)—40 to 60**
4. ***Senium* (extreme old age)—from 60 to death**

Philip de Novare's didactic treatise, *Les Quatre Ages de l'Homme* (c.1260):
1. *Anfance*—from birth to age 20
2. *Jovant*—20 to 40
3. *Moien age* (middle age)—40 to 60
4. ***Viellece* (old age)—60 to 80**

Dante Alighieri's book of verse, *Il Convivio* (c.1304-07):
1. *Adolescenza*—from birth to age 25
2. *Gioventute*—25 to 45
3. **Senetute (old age)—45 to 70**
4. **Senio (extreme old age)—70 to death**

Vincent de Beauvais' scientific encyclopedia, *Speculum Naturale* (1244-54):
1. *Infantia*—birth to age seven
2. *Pueritia*—seven to 14
3. *Adolescentia*—15 to 28
4. *Inventus*—28 to 50
5. **Gravitas (old age)—50 to 72**
6. **Senectus (extreme old age)—72 to death**

Thomas de Cantimpré's scientific encyclopedia, *De Natura Rerum* (c.1228-40):
1. *Infantia*—from birth until the child begins to speak
2. *Pueritia*—from the beginning of speech
3. *Adolescentia*—14 to 35
4. *Robor*—35 to 50
5. **Senectus (old age)—50 to 70**
6. **Etas decrepita (decrepitude)—70 until death**
7. **Mors—death**[199]

NOTES

Introduction

1. Plagues, economic problems, heretical groups, inquisitions, and climatic changes resulting from the 'Little Ice Age' around 1300 (producing a wave of famines, floods, and harvest failures) may have contributed to the rise of witchcraft accusations and trials in the Late Middle Ages, particularly after the fifteenth century (Jeffrey Richards, *Sex, Dissidence and Damnation: Minority Groups in the Middle Ages* (New York: Routledge, 2002), 86). For more information on the growth of witchcraft in the later Middle Ages, see Norman Cohn's *Europe's Inner Demons* and Richard Kieckhefer's *European Witch Trials*.

2. Shulamith Shahar, *Growing Old in the Middle Ages: Winter Clothes Us in Shadow and Pain*, trans. Yael Lotan (New York: Routledge, 2004), 14-15; J. A. Burrow, *The Ages of Man: A Study in Medieval Writing and Thought* (Oxford: Clarendon Press, 1986), 25.

3. Shahar, *Growing Old in the Middle Ages*, 15-17; Marie-Thérèse Lorcin, "Vieillesse et Vieillissment Vus par les Medecins du Moyen Age," *Bulletin du Centre d'Histoire Economique et Sociale de la Region Lyonnaise*, no. 4 (1983): 22. See appendix for the stages of life for the above works.

4. Shahar, *Growing Old in the Middle Ages*, 18; Shahar, "Who were Old in the Middle Ages?," 320.

5. J. B. Post, "Ages at Menarche and Menopause: Some Mediaeval Authorities," *Population Studies* 25, no. 1 (1971): 84; "What is Menopause?," WebMD, http://www.webmd.com.menopause/guide/menopause-basics.

6. Darrel W. Amundsen and Carol Jean Diers, "The Age of Menopause in Medieval Europe," *Human Biology* 45, no. 4 (1973): 607-609.

7. Post, "Ages at Menarche and Menopause," 86.

8. Amundsen and Diers, "The Age of Menopause in Medieval Europe," 609.

9. Albertus Magnus, *Women's Secrets: A Translation of Pseudo-Albertus Magnus's De Secretis Mulierum with Commentaries*, trans. Helen Rodnite LeMay (Albany: State University of New York Press, 1992), 45.

10. Post, "Ages at Menarche and Menopause," 86-87.

Chapter 1. A Time of Change for Women: 1100-1400 in Context

11. Richards, *Sex, Dissidence and Damnation*, 49.

12. Shulamith Shahar, *The Fourth Estate: A History of Women in the Middle Ages*, trans. Chaya Galai (New York: Routledge, 2003), 259.

13. Emmanuel Le Roy Ladurie, *Montaillou: The Promised Land of Error*, trans. Barbara Bray (New York: Vintage Books, 1979), viii; Richards, *Sex, Dissidence and Damnation*, 49-50; Shahar, *The Fourth Estate*, 264.

14. Shahar, *The Fourth Estate*, 259; Richards, *Sex, Dissidence and Damnation*, 49-50.

15. Claire M. Waters, *Angels and Earthly Creatures: Preaching, Performance, and Gender in the Later Middle Ages* (Philadelphia: University of Pennsylvania Press, 2004), 20.

16. Ibid, 20.

17. Jack Holland, *Misogyny: The World's Oldest Prejudice* (New York: Carroll & Graf Publishers, 2006), 105-106, 112; "Twelfth Ecumenical Council: Lateran IV 1215," Internet Medieval Sourcebook, http://www.fordham.edu/halsall/basis/lateran4.html.

18. Shahar, *The Fourth Estate*, 259; Heinrich Fichtenau, *Heretics and Scholars in the High Middle Ages, 1000-1200*, trans. Denise A Kaiser (University Park, Penn: The Pennsylvania State University Press, 1998), 96-97; Michael Costen, *The Cathars and the Albigensian Crusade* (New York: Manchester University Press, 1997), 73, 161.

19. Richards, *Sex, Dissidence and Damnation*, 50-51.

20. Ibid, 55.

21. Ibid, 55-57.

22. Richards, *Sex, Dissidence and Damnation*, 63; Marcia Guttentag and Paul F. Secord, *Too Many Women? The Sex Ratio Question* (Beverly Hills, CA: Sage Publications, Inc., 1983), 63; Shahar, *The Fourth Estate*, 53.

23. Shahar, *The Fourth Estate*, 52-53. The French abbot, chronicler, and poet, Gilles Li Muisis (1272-1352) commented that he only knew the Béguines from hearsay but had heard that they were elderly, wise spinsters (Margaret Wade Labarge, *A Small Sound of the Trumpet: Women in Medieval Life* (Boston: Beacon Press, 1986), 120).

24. Shahar, *The Fourth Estate*, 52-54; Guttentag and Secord, *Too Many Women?*, 63-64; Richards, *Sex, Dissidence and Damnation*, 63.

25. Shahar, *The Fourth Estate*, 54.

26. Guttentag and Secord, *Too Many Women?*, 64.

27. Ibid, 64, 251.

28. Guttentag and Secord, *Too Many Women?*, 63-65; Richards, *Sex, Dissidence and Damnation*, 64. Pope John XXII (1316-1334) later published the Vienne decrees in 1317 (Walter Simons, *Cities of Ladies: Beguine Communities in the Medieval Low Countries, 1200-1565* (Philadelphia: University of Pennsylvania Press, 2001), 133.

29. Simons, *Cities of Ladies*, 133. These heretical beliefs may have included the Béguines' interest in reading religious works in the vernacular, lay preaching, and having a personal relationship with God (Ibid, 141).

30. Ibid, 120, 133.

31. Ibid, 49, 136. In Simons' study of 298 Béguinages in 111 towns and cities in the southern Low Countries between 1200-1565, only four Béguinages are still in existence today (two in Ghent, one in Herentals, and one in Kortrijk) (Ibid, 257-258). For sources, Walter Simons mainly utilized town charters, wills, and tax records.

32. *Manchester Medieval Sources Series: The Black Death*, trans. and ed. Rosemary Horrox (New York: Manchester University Press, 1994), 80-81.

33. Georges Minois, *History of Old Age: From Antiquity to the Renaissance*, trans. Sarah Hanbury Tenison (Chicago: The University of Chicago Press, 1989), 210.

34. Ibid, 210.

35. Minois, *History of Old Age*, 210, 212-213. Demographic data from the High and Late Middle Ages included more men than women since husbands, as heads of households, represented their wives and generally owned more property than women. As a result, there are more names of men in property registers than women (Shahar, *Growing Old in the Middle Ages*, 33-34).

36. Josiah C. Russell, "How Many of the Population were Aged?," in *Aging and the Aged in Medieval Europe: Selected Papers from the Annual Conference of the Centre for Medieval Studies, University of Toronto, held 25-26 February and 11-12 November 1983*, ed. Michael M. Sheehan (Toronto: Pontifical Institute of Mediaeval Studies, 1990), 123-124.

37. Minois, *History of Old Age*, 213.

38. Shahar, *Growing Old in the Middle Ages*, 33-34; David Herlihy, "Life Expectancies for Women in Medieval Society," in *The Role of Woman in the Middle Ages: Papers of the Sixth Annual Conference of the Center for Medieval*

and Early Renaissance Studies, State University of New York at Binghamton, 6-7 May 1972, ed. Rosmarie Thee Morewedge, (Albany: State University of New York Press, 1975), 10-11; Vern Bullough, "Female Longevity and Diet in the Middle Ages," *Speculum* 55, no. 2 (1980): 319-320, 322, 325; Josiah C. Russell, "How Many of the Population were Aged?," 122-123.

39. Herlihy, "Life Expectancies for Women in Medieval Society," 10-11.

40. Judith M. Bennett, *Ale, Beer, and Brewsters in England: Women's Work in a Changing World, 1300-1600* (New York: Oxford University Press, 1996), 114. Bennett states that more sources exist for commercial brewing than for any other female occupation in medieval England since brewing was highly regulated and documented (Ibid, 158).

41. Ibid, 18-19, 24, 27-28. Up until the Black Death in England, brewing was dominated by women. Evidence of this exists in the early twelfth century customs of Newcastle, which employed the word *femina* to describe either a brewer or a baker. In the 1286 charter for Bakewell, Derby, it used the feminine word *pandoxatrix* to describe any ale seller. On most English manors before the plague, mainly women were brought before the court on charges under the assize of ale, which will be fully explained in the main body of the paper (Ibid, 25-26).

42. Ibid, 25-26. Like guilds, freedoms were exclusive memberships to political and economic organizations. In early fourteenth-century Crowle, Lincolnshire, no man was charged as a brewer in the court rolls. On the manors of Brigstock, Ingatestone (Essex), Scalby (Yorkshire), Sutton (Cambridgeshire), and Wakefield, only a few males appeared in the court rolls as brewers during the early fourteenth century. They were usually cited as the husbands of brewsters (Ibid, 25-26).

43. Ibid, 54, 166.

44. Ibid, 99-101.

45. Ibid, 43-44.

46. Ibid, 52.

47. Bennett, *Ale, Beer, and Brewsters in England,* 53-54; Maryanne Kowaleski, "Women's Work in a Market Town: Exeter in the Late Fourteenth Century," in *Women and Work in Preindustrial Europe,* ed. Barbara A. Hanawalt (Bloomington, ID: Indiana University Press, 1986), 150.

48. Bennett, *Ale, Beer, and Brewsters in England,* 51, 174, 178-179.

49. Ibid, 37, 53. In 1381 Southwark, unmarried and widowed brewsters paid considerably less tax than married brewers/brewsters. There were twenty-four brewers/brewsters in Southwark and three were unmarried or widowed. Of the unmarried and widowed, Margery Bruwer paid 4d. in poll tax, Alice Jolyf

paid 12d., and Joan Saunders paid 12d. William Weston and his wife were taxed 5s. and so were Thomas Hosyar and his wife, and ten other couples were charged between 3 and 4s. (Ibid, 53).

50. Ibid. 113-114.

Chapter 2. Didactic and Prescriptive Works on Old Age

51. Hildegard of Bingen, *Selected Writings*, trans. Mark Atherton (New York: Penguin Books, 2001), 6, 253.

52. Ibid, 6.

53. Roger Bacon, *The Opus Majus of Roger Bacon*, vol. 1, trans. Robert Belle Burke (New York: Russell & Russell Inc., 1962), xi.

54. Bacon, *The Opus Majus*, vol. 2, 619.

55. Ibid, 619. In Bacon's description concerning old age, he did not specify whether he was representing old men or women.

56. Shaher, *Growing Old in the Middle Ages*, 38.

57. Bacon, *Opus Majus*, vol. 2, 619.

58. In Aristotle's *Politics*, he compared old people to children: "An old person and a young person are born incomplete in mind and body, while people in old age are weak. Their mind is no longer prime when they are old". *The Politics* was first translated into Latin in the mid-thirteenth century (Aristotle, *The Politics*, trans. Carnes Lord (Chicago: University of Chicago Press, 1984), 224, 226).

59. Elizabeth Joy Keen, *The Journey of a Book: Bartholomew the Englishman and the Properties of Things* (Canberra, AU: E Press, 2007), 4-5. There are over two hundred manuscripts of *On the Properties of Things* in existence.

60. Lorcin, "Vieillesse et Vieillissement," 7. Bartholomaeus Anglicus was referring to all old people - male and female.

61. Philippe de Navarre, *Les Quatre Ages de l'Homme*, ed. Marcel de Fréville (New York: Johnson Reprint Corporation, 1968), XIV-XVIII.

62. Karen Pratt, "De Vetula: The Figure of the Old Woman in Medieval French Literature," in *Old Age in the Middle Ages and the Renaissance: Interdisciplinary Approaches to a Neglected Topic*, ed. Albrecht Classen (New York: Walter de Gruyter, 2007), 324. In Philip de Novare's description regarding old age, he did not specify whether he was depicting middle-aged men or women.

63. Shahar, *Growing Old in the Middle Ages*, 15-16; Pratt, "De Vetula," 325.

64. Andreas Capellanus, *The Art of Courtly Love*, trans. John Jay Parry (New York: Columbia University Press, 1960), 17.

65. Ibid, 21-22.

66. Ibid, 32.

67. Herbert C. Covey, "Perceptions and Attitudes Toward Sexuality of the Elderly During the Middle Ages," *The Gerontologist* 29, no. 1 (1989): 95. The idea of love ending at menopause was not a new concept during the Middle Ages. In Aristotle's *Masterpiece*, he stated that sexual activity and desire ended for women at menopause. *Masterpiece* was a very popular reference book on sex and reproduction throughout the medieval period (Ibid, 95).

68. Pratt, "De Vetula," 325-326; Shahar, *Growing Old in the Middles Ages*, 78-79.

69. Ibid, 94-96, 99.

70. Albertus Magnus, *Women's Secrets*, 1, 50. There are currently eighty-three manuscripts of *De Secretis Mulierum* in existence.

71. Shaher, *Growing Old in the Middle Ages*, 44.

72. Ibid, 44.

73. Albertus Magnus, *Women's Secrets*, 129-131.

74. Ibid, 129-130.

75. Ibid, 22, 35, 37, 48-49.

Chapter 3. Old Women in Literature

76. Derek Pearsall, *The Canterbury Tales* (Boston: George Allen & Unwin, 1985), 8.

77. Geoffrey Chaucer, *The Canterbury Tales* (New York: Random House, 1965), 174-175, 176.

78. Ibid, 176.

79. Ibid, 181.

80. William Calin, *The French Tradition and the Literature of Medieval England* (Buffalo: University of Toronto Press, 1994), 331; Chaucer, *The Canterbury Tales* (1965), 177, 183.

81. Chaucer, *The Canterbury Tales* (1965), 177, 181-182.

82. Calin, *The French Tradition*, 331, Chaucer, *The Canterbury Tales* (1965), 182, 184.

83. Chaucer, *The Canterbury Tales* (1965), 182, 184, 187-188.

84. Ibid, 197.

85. Minois, *History of Old Age*, 226-227; *The Fifteen Joys of Marriage*, trans. Brent A. Pitts (New York: Peter Lang Publishing, 1985), 116-117; Melinda Marsh Heywood, *Lady Philosophy and La Vieille: Old Women, Aging Bodies, and Female Authority in Late Medieval French Literature* (Ann Arbor, MI: UMI, 1997), 124-125. The author of *The Fifteen Joys of Marriage* is unknown. The author of *The Fifteen Joys of Marriage* explained that young men typically married old women out of avarice and never out of love (Minois, *History of Old Age*, 226).

86. Minois, *History of Old Age*, 226.

87. Heywood, *Lady Philosophy and La Vieille*, 125; Lois Banner, *In Full Flower: Aging Women, Power and Sexuality* (New York: Alfred A. Knopf, 1992), 155; Robert Magnan, "Sex and Senescence in Medieval Literature," in *Aging in Literature*, ed. Laurel Porter and Laurence M. Porter (Troy, MI: International Book Publishers, 1984), 13.

88. Heywood, *Lady Philosophy and La Vieille*, 125. Jean Le Fèvre translated *Liber lamentationum Matheoluli* into French around c. 1371-1372 (Alcuin Blamires, Karen Pratt, and C. W. Marx, ed., *Woman Defamed and Woman Defended: An Anthology of Medieval Texts* (Oxford: Clarendon Press, 1992), 177).

89. *Lyrics of the Troubadours and Trouvères: An Anthology and a History*, trans. Frederick Goldin (New York: Anchor Books, 1973), 333. The main difference between the troubadours and the trouvères is that the troubadours were from southern France while the trouvères were from northern France.

90. Ibid, 345. This quote resembles a quote from Aristophanes' *Lysistrata*: "A man comes home - he may be old and grey - but he can get himself a wife in no time. But a woman's not in bloom for long, and if she doesn't succeed quickly, there's no one will marry her, and before long she's going round to the fortune tellers to ask them is she's any chance" (Minois, *History of Old Age*, 53). So, a man can get married at any age, while a woman's chances of marriage declines with age.

91. Ibid, 347.

92. Guillaume de Lorris and Jean de Meun, *The Romance of the Rose*, trans. Charles Dahlberg (Princeton, NJ: Princeton University Press, 1971), 1-2; Calin, *The French Tradition*, 161. Over three hundred manuscripts of *The Romance of the Rose* exist.

93. De Lorris and De Meun, *The Romance of the Rose*, 223, 225.

94. Calin, *The French Tradition*, 327-328; De Lorris and De Meun, *The Romance of the Rose*, 226-227, 246-247.

95. De Lorris and De Meun, *The Romance of the Rose*, 222, 247.

96. Ibid, 222-223, 247-248.

97. Ibid, 222.

98. Calin, *The French Tradition*, 328.

99. Blamires, Pratt, and Marx, *Woman Defamed and Woman Defended*, 21-23.

100. *Seven Medieval Latin Comedies*, trans. Alison Goddard Elliott (New York: Garland Publishing, Inc., 1984), xxvi, xxxiii. By 1610, there were sixteen printed editions (first edition was printed by 1470) of *Pamphilus*.

101. Ibid, 6.

102. Ibid, 7-8.

103. Ibid, 9.
104. Ibid, 2, 11.
105. Ibid, 19-20.
106. Ibid, 20-21.
107. Ibid, 21, 24.
108. Ibid, 20-21.
109. Ibid, 22-23.
110. Ibid, 23.
111. Ibid, 24.
112. Giovanni Boccaccio, *Il Filocolo*, trans. Donald Cheney and Thomas G. Bergin (New York: Garland Publishing, Inc., 1985), xii-xiii.
113. Ibid, 290.
114. Ibid, 291.
115. Ibid, 291.
116. Ibid, 291-292.
117. A. C. Cawley, ed., *Pearl/Sir Gawain and the Green Knight* (New York: E. P. Dutton & Co. Inc., 1962), 86-87. The author(s) of the poem, "Sir Gawain and the Green Knight" is unknown.
118. Ibid, 87.
119. Ibid, 86-87.
120. Ibid, 27.
121. Ibid, 143.
122. Jonathan H. Hsy, "John Gower: Life, Work, and Times," John Gower Webpage, http://home.gwu.edu/~jhsy/gower.html.; John Gower, *Confessio Amantis*, trans. Terence Tiller (Baltimore, MD: Penguin Books, 1963), 12; John Gower, *Confessio Amantis*, ed. Russell A. Peck (New York: Holt, Rinehart & Winston, 1968), xxxii.
123. Chaucer, *The Canterbury Tales* (1965), 190-191, Gower, *Confessio Amantis* (1968), 58-60.
124. Chaucer, *The Canterbury Tales* (1965), 192.
125. Gower, *Confessio Amantis* (1963), 70-71.
126. Chaucer, *The Canterbury Tales* (1965), 192.
127. Gower, *Confessio Amantis* (1968), 62; Chaucer, *The Canterbury Tales* (1965), 192-193.
128. Gower, *Confessio Amantis* (1968), 62-63, 65; Chaucer, *The Canterbury Tales* (1965), 193.
129. Chaucer, *The Canterbury Tales* (1965), 194, 196.
130. Ibid, 196. In Gower's version, the old woman gave him the choice of having her old and ugly by day and young and beautiful at night or the reverse (Gower, *Confessio Amantis* (1963), 70).

131. Ibid, 196.

132. Ibid, 196-197.

133. Chaucer, *The Canterbury Tales* (1965), 145.

134. Ibid, 145.

135. Ibid, 204-205. A harridan is a shrew.

136. Ibid, 204.

137. Ibid, 205.

138. Ibid, 205.

139. Wolfram von Eschenbach, *Willehalm*, trans. Marion E. Gibbs and Sidney M. Johnson (New York: Penguin Books, 1984), 230, 268.

140. Ibid, 88.

141. Ibid, 88.

142. Ibid, 88.

143. Ibid, 119-120.

144. Ibid, 120.

145. Giovanni Boccaccio, *The Decameron*, vol. 1 of *The Tudor Translations* (New York: AMS Press Inc., 1967), cxix. In fact, Geoffrey Chaucer translated parts of *The Decameron* - the first story of the eighth day, the fifth story of the tenth day, and the tenth story of the tenth day (Ibid, cxxii).

146. Giovanni Boccaccio, *The Decameron*, trans. John Payne (New York: Liveright Publishing Corp, 1943), 366-367.

147. St. Thomas Aquinas (1225-1274) regarded women as a "man's helpmate" who are "needed to preserve the species or to provide food and drink" (Holland, *Misogyny*, 112). Once again, women are confined to only two roles - having children and providing nourishment.

148. Boccaccio, *The Decameron* (1943), 367. The association between a woman's worth and her reproductive ability was apparent in the Book of Leviticus and the wergeld system during the Early Middle Ages. The Book of Leviticus included laws where a person promised to offer God the value of another. In the Book of Leviticus (27:1-7), the value of a woman between twenty to sixty years of age was valued at thirty shekels. At sixty, a woman was valued at ten shekels, the same as a girl between five to twenty years of age. The wergeld compensated families whose relations had been killed. In the wergeld system under the Visogoths, a woman between fifteen to forty years of age was worth two hundred and fifty solidi. A woman between forty to sixty years was worth two hundred solidi and a woman over sixty was worth one hundred solidi (Shahar, *Growing Old in the Middle Ages*, 5-6). Under the law of the Salian Franks, a young girl was worth two hundred solidi, a woman in her childbearing years was valued at six hundred solidi, a pregnant woman was

valued at seven hundred solidi, and an old woman was worth two hundred solidi (Herlihy, "Life Expectancies for Women in Medieval Society," 8-9). From these figures, it can be suggested that a woman's value declined as her economic and reproductive abilities diminished.

149. Boccaccio, *The Decameron* (1943), 367.

Chapter 4. The Lives of Post-Menopausal Women in the High and Late Middle Ages

150. Barbara Newman, "Sibyl of the Rhine: Hildegard's Life and Times," in *Voice of the Living Light: Hildegard of Bingen and Her World*, ed. Barbara Newman (Los Angeles: University of California Press, 1998), 12; John Van Engen, "Abbess: Mother and Teacher," in *Voice of the Living Light: Hildegard of Bingen and Her World*, ed. Barbara Newman (Los Angeles: University of California Press, 1998), 30, 40; Hildegard of Bingen, *Selected Writings*, 243.

151. Newman, "Sibyl of the Rhine," 22; Hildegard of Bingen, *Selected Writings*, liii-liv.

152. Newman, "Sibyl of the Rhine," 22; Van Engen, "Abbess," 30. Hildegard brought eighteen nuns with her when she founded the convent at Rupertsberg. By the time of Hildegard's death, the convent accommodated up to fifty nuns (Newman, "Sibyl of the Rhine," 14; Van Engen, "Abbess: Mother and Teacher," 30).

153. Marjorie Chibnall, *The Empress Matilda: Queen Consort, Queen Mother and Lady of the English* (Cambridge, MA: Blackwell, 1991), 159, 161. Matilda's first husband was Henry V, emperor of Germany, and her second husband was Geoffrey, count of Anjou, who was the father of Henry II.

154. Ibid, 158-160-186. Robert of Torigny's *Chronicle* recorded the reigns of Stephen of Blois, Henry II, and Richard I.

155. Ibid, 159-160, 162-163, 186-189.

156. Alison Weir, *Eleanor of Aquitaine: A Life* (New York: Ballantine Books, 1999), 180, 196, 202, 211. Crowning an heir to the throne during a father's lifetime was a French tradition introduced by Charlemagne. Henry II wanted to bring this custom to England in order to secure royal succession. After the coronation ceremony, Henry's son was known as Henry the Young King (Ibid, 179).

157. Peter of Blois, "Letter 154 to Queen Eleanor of Aquitaine, 1173," Internet Medieval Sourcebook, http://www.fordham.edu/halsall/source/eleanor.html.

158. Weir, *Eleanor of Aquitaine*, 211.

159. Shahar, *Growing Old in the Middle Ages*, 126; Weir, *Eleanor of Aquitaine*, 260-261.

160. Amy Kelly, *Eleanor of Aquitaine and the Four Kings* (Cambridge, Mass: Harvard University Press, 1978), 263-264.

161. Weir, *Eleanor of Aquitaine*, 260.

162. LaBarge, *A Small Sound of the Trumpet*, 51-52; Weir, *Eleanor of* Aquitaine, 250, 281.

163. Shahar, *Growing Old in the Middle Ages*, 126.

164. Weir, *Eleanor of Aquitaine*, 301, 313, 317; Shahar, *Growing Old in the Middle Ages*, 126.

165. LaBarge, *A Small Sound of the Trumpet*, 52; Shahar, *Growing Old in the Middle Ages*, 126; Weir, *Eleanor of Aquitaine*, 330.

166. LaBarge, *A Small Sound of the Trumpet*, 52-55. Blanche died while Louis IX was on crusade (Ibid, 55).

167. Ibid, 55.

168. Shahar, *Growing Old in the Middle Ages*, 127; LaBarge, *A Small Sound of the Trumpet*, 81-82; Karen S. Nicholas, "Countesses as Rulers in Flanders," in *Aristocratic Women in Medieval France*, ed. Theodore Evergates (Philadelphia: University of Pennsylvania Press, 1999), 133-135.

169. Emmanuel Le Roy Ladurie, *Montaillou*, 166-167. Le Roy Ladurie's sources for *Montaillou* came from interrogations conducted by the papal Inquisition under Bishop Jacques Fournier of Pamiers between 1318-1325. Twenty-five of the accused and several witnesses from Montaillou were interrogated before the Inquisition. The population of Montaillou during this time was around 200-250 (Ibid, xiv, 3).

170. Le Roy Ladurie, *Montaillou*, 3, 167, xiii-xiv; Banner, *In Full Flower*, 162-163.

171. Béatrice and Barthélemy would meet again in 1320 when she asked him to help her escape from the Inquisition. She planned to flee Jacques Fournier's summons by hiding out at her sister's house in Limoux. On their way to Limoux, Béatrice and Barthélemy were caught and arrested by Fournier's associates. They were interrogated by Fournier and imprisoned at Allemans until they were released on 4 July 1322. Béatrice's prison sentence was commuted to wearing two yellow crosses on her clothing, while Barthélemy walked free from prison with minor penances (René Weis, *The Yellow Cross: The Story of the Last Cathars, 1290-1329* (New York: Alfred A. Knopf, 2001), 321-323, 363).

172. Le Roy Ladurie, *Montaillou*, 168.

173. Barbara A. Hanawalt, *The Ties That Bound: Peasant Families in Medieval England* (New York: Oxford University Press, 1986), 237-238, 39.

174. Barbara Hanawalt, "Remarriage as an Option for Urban and Rural Widows in Late Medieval England," in *Wife and Widow in Medieval England*, ed. Sue Sheridan Walker (Ann Arbor, MI: University of Michigan Press, 1993), 141; Hanawalt, *The Ties That Bound*, 220.

175. Hanawalt, "Remarriage as an Option," 144; Shahar, *Growing Old in the Middle Ages*, 128; Judith M. Bennett, *Women in the Medieval English Countryside: Gender and Household in Brigstock Before the Plague* (New York: Oxford University Press, 1987), 163.

176. Shahar, *Growing Old in the Middle Ages*, 126-127.

177. Shahar, *Growing Old in the Middle Ages*, 156; Hanawalt, *The Ties That Bound*, 221.

178. Hanawalt, *The Ties That Bound*, 221-222.

179. Hanawalt, *The Ties That Bound*, 236; Shahar, *Growing Old in the Middle Ages*, 144.

180. Bennett, *Women in the Medieval English* Countryside, 151. For primary sources, Bennett mainly used manorial court rolls dating from February 1287 to September 1348.

181. Bennett, *Women in the Medieval English Countryside*, 151, 159, 172, 164-165. Younger widows with young children were more likely to remarry than older widows. Also, when land was readily available, as in Brigstock, widows remarried less. Retirement provisions included maintenance agreements in which widows gave away property (usually to sons) in exchange for support (Ibid, 61, 146-147).

182. The exact ages of the following widows are unknown. Their ages can only be estimated by their (average) age at marriage, their length of marriage, and their length of widowhood. The average age at marriage for peasants during the fourteenth century was between eighteen and twenty-two years old. The average duration of marriage in Brigstock was around twenty years (Ibid, 72, 143).

183. Ibid, 152, 158-159.

184. Ibid, 151, 155, 158.

185. Ibid, 142-143.

186. Ibid, 148-149. A pledger was a person who made sure that one met their legal obligations. The five men made a total of twenty-six court appearances as pledgers and officers in the first decade, one hundred and seventy-six appearances in the second decade, one hundred and seventy-two appearances

in the third decade, one hundred and twenty-seven appearances in the fourth decade, and ten appearances in the fifth decade (Ibid, 148).

187. Ibid, 147.
188. Le Roy Ladurie, *Montaillou*, 190, 216. The case of Montaillou shows us one pattern of society. One should not make generalizations on this one model alone.
189. Ibid, 216.
190. Shahar, *Growing Old in the Middle Ages*, 152.
191. Le Roy Ladurie, *Montaillou*, 34, 216-217.
192. Ibid, 196.
193. Shahar, *Growing Old in the Middle Ages*, 127.
194. Ibid, 151.
195. Shahar, *Growing Old in the Middle Ages*, 150; Banner, *In Full Flower*, 161; Le Roy Ladurie, *Montaillou*, 194, 196-197.
196. Le Roy Ladurie, *Montaillou*, 196, 222, 251, 367.

Appendix

197. Shahar, *Growing Old in the Middle Ages*, 15.
198. Lorcin, "Vieillesse et Vieillissment Vus par les Medecins du Moyen Age," 22.
199. Shahar, *Growing Old in the Middle Ages*, 15-17.

BIBLIOGRAPHY

Primary Sources

Albertus Magnus. *Women's Secrets: A Translation of Pseudo-Albertus Magnus's De Secretis Mulierum with Commentaries.* Translated by Helen Rodnite LeMay. Albany: State University of New York Press, 1992.

Andreas Capellanus. *The Art of Courtly Love.* Translated by John Jay Parry. New York: Columbia University Press, 1960.

Aristotle. *The Politics.* Translated by Carnes Lord. Chicago: University of Chicago Press, 1984.

Bacon, Roger. *The Opus Majus of Roger Bacon.* 2 vols. Translated by Robert Belle Burke. New York: Russell & Russell Inc., 1962.

Blamires, Alcuin, Karen Pratt, and C. W. Marx, ed. *Woman Defamed and Woman Defended: An Anthology of Medieval Texts.* Oxford: Clarendon Press, 1992.

Boccaccio, Giovanni. *The Decameron.* Translated by John Payne. New York: Liveright Publishing Corp, 1943.

_____. *The Decameron.* Vol. 1, *The Tudor Translations.* New York: AMS Press Inc., 1967.

_____. *Il Filocolo.* Translated by Donald Cheney and Thomas G. Bergin. New York: Garland Publishing, Inc., 1985.

Cawley, A. C., ed. *Pearl/Sir Gawain and the Green Knight*. New York: E. P. Dutton & Co. Inc., 1962.

Chaucer, Geoffrey. *The Canterbury Tales*. New York: Random House, 1965.

The Fifteen Joys of Marriage. Translated by Brent A. Pitts. New York: Peter Lang Publishing, 1985.

Gower, John. *Confessio Amantis*. Edited by Russell A. Peck. New York: Holt, Rinehart & Winston, 1968.

_____. *Confessio Amantis*. Translated by Terence Tiller. Baltimore, MD: Penguin Books, 1963.

Hildegard of Bingen. *Selected Writings*. Translated by Mark Atherton. New York: Penguin Books, 2001.

Lorris, Guillaume de, and Jean de Meun. *The Romance of the Rose*. Translated by Charles Dahlberg. Princeton, NJ: Princeton University Press, 1971.

Lyrics of the Troubadours and Trouveres: An Anthology and a History. Translated by Frederick Goldin. New York: Anchor Books, 1973.

Manchester Medieval Sources Series: The Black Death. Translated and Edited by Rosemary Horrox. New York: Manchester University Press, 1994.

Peter of Blois. "Letter 154 to Queen Eleanor of Aquitaine, 1173." Internet Medieval Sourcebook. http://www.fordham.edu/halsall/source/eleanor.html.

Philippe de Navarre. *Les Quatre Ages de l'Homme*. Edited by Marcel de Fréville. New York: Johnson Reprint Corporation, 1968.

Seven Medieval Latin Comedies. Translated by Alison Goddard Elliott. New York: Garland Publishing, Inc., 1984.

"Twelfth Ecumenical Council: Lateran IV 1215." Internet Medieval Sourcebook. http://www.fordham.edu/halsall/basis/lateran4.html.

Secondary Sources

Amundsen, Darrel W., and Carol Jean Diers. "The Age of Menopause in Medieval Europe." *Human Biology* 45, no. 4 (1973): 605-612.

Banner, Lois W. *In Full Flower: Aging Women, Power and Sexuality.* New York: Alfred A. Knopf, 1992.

Bennett, Judith M. *Ale, Beer, and Brewsters in England: Women's Work in a Changing World, 1300-1600.* New York: Oxford University Press, 1996.

_____. *Women in the Medieval English Countryside: Gender and Household in Brigstock Before the Plague.* New York: Oxford University Press, 1987.

Burrow, J. A. *The Ages of Man: A Study in Medieval Writing and Thought.* Oxford: Clarendon Press, 1986.

Calin, William. *The French Tradition and the Literature of Medieval England.* Buffalo: University of Toronto Press, 1994.

Chibnall, Marjorie. *The Empress Matilda: Queen Consort, Queen Mother and Lady of the English.* Cambridge, MA: Blackwell, 1991.

Classen, Albrecht, ed. *Old Age in the Middle Ages and the Renaissance: Interdisciplinary Approaches to a Neglected Topic.* New York: Walter de Gruyter, 2007.

Costen, Michael. *The Cathars and the Albigensian Crusade.* New York: Manchester University Press, 1997.

Covey, Herbert C. "Perceptions and Attitudes Toward Sexuality of the Elderly During the Middle Ages." *The Gerontologist* 29, no. 1 (1989): 93-100.

Ferrante, Joan. "Correspondent." In *Voice of the Living Light: Hildegard of Bingen and Her World,* edited by Barbara Newman, 91-109. Los Angeles: University of California Press, 1998.

Fichtenau, Heinrich. *Heretics and Scholars in the High Middle Ages, 1000-1200*. Translated by Denise A Kaiser. University Park, PA: The Pennsylvania State University Press, 1998.

Guttentag, Marcia, and Paul F. Secord. *Too Many Women? The Sex Ratio Question*. Beverly Hills, CA: Sage Publications, Inc., 1983.

Hanawalt, Barbara A. "Remarriage as an Option for Urban and Rural Widows in Late Medieval England." In *Wife and Widow in Medieval England*, edited by Sue Sheridan Walker, 141-164. Ann Arbor, MI: University of Michigan Press, 1993.

_____. *The Ties That Bound: Peasant Families in Medieval England*. New York: Oxford University Press, 1986.

Herlihy, David. "Life Expectancies for Women in Medieval Society." In *The Role of Woman in the Middle Ages: Papers of the Sixth Annual Conference of the Center for Medieval and Early Renaissance Studies, State University of New York at Binghamton, 6-7 May 1972*, edited by Rosmarie Thee Morewedge, 1-22. Albany: State University of New York Press, 1975.

Heywood, Melinda Marsh. *Lady Philosophy and La Vieille: Old Women, Aging Bodies, and Female Authority in Late Medieval French Literature*. Ann Arbor, MI: UMI, 1997.

Holland, Jack. *Misogyny: The World's Oldest Prejudice*. New York: Carroll & Graf Publishers, 2006.

Hsy, Jonathan H. "John Gower: Life, Work, and Times." John Gower Webpage. http://home.gwu.edu/~jhsy/gower.html.

Keen, Elizabeth Joy. *The Journey of a Book: Bartholomew the Englishman and the Properties of Things*. Canberra, AU: E Press, 2007.

Kelly, Amy. *Eleanor of Aquitaine and the Four Kings*. Cambridge, Mass: Harvard University Press, 1978.

Kowaleski, Maryanne. "Women's Work in a Market Town: Exeter in the Late Fourteenth Century." In *Women and Work in Preindustrial Europe*, edited by Barbara A. Hanawalt, 145-164. Bloomington, ID: Indiana University Press, 1986.

LaBarge, Margaret Wade. *A Small Sound of the Trumpet: Women in Medieval Life*. Boston: Beacon Press, 1986.

Le Roy Ladurie, Emmanuel. *Montaillou: The Promised Land of Error*. Translated by Barbara Bray. New York: Vintage Books, 1979.

Lorcin, Marie-Thérèse. "Vieillesse et Vieillissment Vus par les Medecins du Moyen Age." *Bulletin du Centre d'Histoire Economique et Sociale de la Region Lyonnaise*, no. 4 (1983): 5-22.

Magnan, Robert. "Sex and Senescence in Medieval Literature." In *Aging in Literature*, edited by Laurel Porter and Laurence M. Porter, 13-30. Troy, MI: International Book Publishers, 1984.

Minois, Georges. *History of Old Age: From Antiquity to the Renaissance*. Translated by Sarah Hanbury Tenison. Chicago: The University of Chicago Press, 1989.

Newman, Barbara. "Sibyl of the Rhine: Hildegard's Life and Times." In *Voice of the Living Light: Hildegard of Bingen and Her World*, edited by Barbara Newman, 1-29. Los Angeles: University of California Press, 1998.

Nicholas, Karen S. "Countesses as Rulers in Flanders." In *Aristocratic Women in Medieval France*, edited by Theodore Evergates, 111-137. Philadelphia: University of Pennsylvania Press, 1999.

Pearsall, Derek. *The Canterbury Tales*. Boston: George Allen & Unwin, 1985.

Post, J. B. "Ages at Menarche and Menopause: Some Mediaeval Authorities." *Population Studies* 25, no. 1 (1971): 83-87.

Pratt, Karen. "De Vetula: The Figure of the Old Woman in Medieval French Literature." In *Old Age in the Middle Ages and the Renaissance: Interdisciplinary Approaches to a Neglected Topic*, edited by Albrecht Classen, 321-342. New York: Walter de Gruyter, 2007.

Richards, Jeffrey. *Sex, Dissidence and Damnation: Minority Groups in the Middle Ages*. New York: Routledge, 2002.

Russell, Josiah C. "How Many of the Population were Aged?" In *Aging and the Aged in Medieval Europe: Selected Papers from the Annual Conference of the Centre for Medieval Studies, University of Toronto, held 25-26 February and 11-12 November 1983*, edited by Michael M. Sheehan, 119-127. Toronto: Pontifical Institute of Mediaeval Studies, 1990.

Shahar, Shulamith. *The Fourth Estate: A History of Women in the Middle Ages*. Translated by Chaya Galai. New York: Routledge, 2003.

_____. *Growing Old in the Middle Ages: Winter Clothes Us in Shadow and Pain*. Translated by Yael Lotan. New York: Routledge, 2004.

_____. "Who were Old in the Middle Ages?" *Social History of Medicine* 6, no. 3 (1993): 313-341.

Van Engen, John. "Abbess: Mother and Teacher." In *Voice of the Living Light: Hildegard of Bingen and Her World*, edited by Barbara Newman, 30-51. Los Angeles: University of California Press, 1998.

Waters, Claire M. *Angels and Earthly Creatures: Preaching, Performance, and Gender in the Later Middle Ages*. Philadelphia: University of Pennsylvania Press, 2004.

Weir, Alison. *Eleanor of Aquitaine: A Life*. New York: Ballantine Books, 1999.

Weis, René. *The Yellow Cross: The Story of the Last Cathars, 1290-1329*. New York: Alfred A. Knopf, 2001.

"What is Menopause?" WebMD. http://www.webmd.com.menopause/guide/menopause-basics.